RECLAIM YOUR HEALTH

Learn how to overcome the most common chronic illnesses

CARDIOVASCULAR DISEASES

By Award Winning Author
DR HARRIS PHILLIP

Disclaimer

The publisher and authors are not responsible for any specific health needs that may require medical supervision. If you have underlying health problems or have any doubts about the advice contained in this book, please contact a qualified medical doctor or an appropriately trained healthcare professional. It is not intended as, and should not be relied upon as, medical advice despite having an author with 30+ years' experience in practice in the medical field.

The information contained within this book series, Reclaim Your Health: learn how to overcome the 9 most common chronic health challenges in modern times, Cardiovascular Diseases is not intended to be used in the place of your general practitioner's advice or your family doctor's advice. This book series is provided for general information only and to empower readers by providing them with relevant information on the disease in an easily digestible format, thus ensuring their visits with their healthcare professional are richer and more rewarding. It will go a long way in helping you understand the pathognomonic features of this commonly seen chronic conditions called cardiovascular diseases, and it will provide you with some usable tools which you can employ to protect yourself from the daily insults on our bodies.

CONTENTS

Foreword

By Professor Ali Nakash

While continuing with his 30+ years' experience in clinical practice, Harris has decided to sum up much of what he has gained from seeing and treating thousands, maybe millions, of patients with a myriad of medical problems over the years. In his summary, which has been compiled into a series of twelve chunk-sized books, the reader is provided with usable tools which are presented in a simple, readily digestible format to allow everyone to benefit. From the least medically inclined among us, to the nursing student, the pharmacy student, the nurse, the pharmacist, the midwifery student, the midwife, the medical student, and the trained doctor, whether junior or senior. In essence there are useful nuggets of easy-to-follow guidance for all.

In the first book in the series, he starts with a disease we all dread. Many including my wife call it that disease…. You certainly know the disease to which I refer, it is cancer.

Reading through the pages of the first book in this series, I was immediately impressed with the presentation. Such a complex condition was condensed into such simple and easy-to-follow guidance. Not only has he addressed cancer from its cellular level, but he has also extended the discussion to allow you, the reader, to appreciate plausible causative agents for this condition once it is initiated. He gives some insight into how the disease process flourishes, and towards the end of the book he addresses how we can make ourselves cancer-proof.

Making ourselves cancer-proof I find particularly interesting since it allows both medical and non-medical personnel to explore avenues through which they can empower both themselves and their patients as together we fight this dreaded disease.

In the other books of this series which are being completed, the approach is the same, whether it is addressing Alzheimer's disease, cardiovascular disease, diabetes, or the other chronic health challenges of our time. I am particularly impressed with the presentation, the relative simplicity, and the inherent usefulness of this series. This doubtlessly will not only empower, but also serve as a useful companion handbook on our journey to reclaiming our health.

Mr. Phillip is an award-winning author for his book, STOP! It's Not Too Late!: Adding Years to Your Life and Life to Your Years Using the BMS Model, a book which I call an encyclopaedic guide to healthy living. But in this book series I think he has outdone himself as he seeks to provide the tools that we all need to reclaim our health.

He has most definitely put his years of training and experience in capsule form through the various books in this series. Mr Phillip is a trained senior consultant obstetrician and gynaecologist and has displayed his abundance of knowledge through the ease with which he addresses the various chronic health challenges of our times.

This series, for me, represents an interesting and empowering piece of medical science which has been presented in a digestible format for even the non-medical personnel among us. I am therefore moved to make this bold prediction that once you start reading these books, you will find it difficult to stop because of the timeliness and appropriateness of their contents.

Introduction

Several years ago, I was employed as a teacher, which incidentally was my first professional job. While entering the classroom to deliver a biology lecture to a group of students at the Saint Andrews High School, who were preparing to write the General Certificate of Education examination (GCE or GCSE, as referred to in the UK), a young man who claimed he had no interest in Biology collected his books and was leaving the classroom to go to the library, as I entered to deliver the lecture. The lecture was designed to highlight the characteristics of living things and to help distinguish the living from the dead. I commenced the lecture with the statement, 'once one starts living, he/she starts dying'. Inherent in that statement is that both living and dying are processes. Even deeper is the realisation that what we refer to as life is simply a grant of two dates and a dash. Upon hearing this introduction, the young man made an about-turn and asked permission to attend my class. I did not convert him into a biologist, but he left the class much better informed. Today that young man is a politician. We are granted a date of birth and a date of death: between these two dates is the dash and that is the focus of this book, how can we extend the dash to delay our date of death. I prefer to look at the whole scenario as a rubber band that can be stretched between two points, the two points being the date of birth and the date of death. We can do nothing about our date of birth, that date is beyond our control, but if my analogy of a rubber band is fully understood, and since our date of birth cannot be seriously influenced by our action or inaction, for the rubber band concept to hold, it means that the dash can be extended and thus we can delay our date of death.

My paternal grandmother, for instance, lived to a ripe old age of 115 years. She lived a fully independent life, still being able to cook and care for herself in her 115th year. This is not widespread, I hear you say, and my response is why not? Do we have any skills, knowledge, or abilities in the current era to approach this lifespan and make it more of the expected norm as opposed to an occasional event?

It is with this burning desire that I have used my medical knowledge, gleaned in the field, as well as my extensive research, the skills of which I learned as a university student in organic and biochemistry at a top 10 USA university as I pursed a PhD degree in Biochemistry. This training not only provided me with the skills and tools which I needed to pursue the more inquisitive aspect of my person, but also has alerted me to the value of research. Thus, when faced with a challenging question, I revert to research to help me determine the answer.

In observing the lifestyle of my paternal grandmother, my 30+ years of medical practice, drawing on the knowledge gleaned through my research, and from my study in organic chemistry, leading to my Master's degree and my sojourn through the biochemistry classroom, I believe that we have an opportunity to delay the second date, the date of death, by stretching in rubber band style the duration of the dash. This is therefore the purpose of this book: providing tools, suggestions and basic information which will hopefully allow you to prolong your dash and live a more dynamic and healthier lifestyle, thus adding years to your life and life to your years.

I will aim to provide sections on each of the nine most common chronic ailments of our time, suggesting how best one can delay the effect of the insult on our bodies, hence allowing us to live a more complete, fun-filled life, a guide to which has been developed in one of my earlier books, about using the BMS approach, an award-winning book.

In this book series we will look at cancer, Alzheimer's, dementia and diseases of the brain, heart disease and strokes, diabetes, arthritis, obesity, chronic lung diseases, and chronic kidney diseases, hoping that this serves as a useful handbook – guide, if you will – in understanding and defeating the most common chronic ailments affecting human beings on planet earth.

I know that you may be stunned: why has a trained obstetrician and gynaecologist got involved in the writing of books addressing various aspects of health, some of which may be remote from obstetrics (care of pregnant ladies during their pregnancy and childbirth and for the first 42 days after ending the pregnancy) and gynaecology (the branch of medicine which deals with the functions and diseases specific to women and girls, specifically those relating to the reproductive system)? To this my response is simple:

It is the only medical discipline which allows one to practise all the facets of medicine. It therefore means that any good obstetrician and gynaecologist, because of the demands on his scope of practice, needs to be above average in his knowledge of internal medicine, surgery, paediatrics, social and preventative medicine, care of the elderly, and neonatology. Hence my familiarity with these various disciplines and the related physiology has empowered me in the provision of this book series which I am hopeful will be an empowering tool to help many understand elements of their health, while simultaneously allowing them to know when things are wrong and therefore see the need to seek medical advice. Hopefully the message is that the earlier a disease process is found, the more options will be available for management and the more likely a full cure will be realised.

BOOK 3
CARDIOVASCULAR DISEASE

CHAPTER 1
Cardiovascular Health

- Why

- The meaning of cardiovascular health

  o Suggestion 1

  o Suggestion 2

  o Suggestion 3

  o Suggestion 4

  o Suggestion 5

- Statins and the cholesterol story

- Statins rob our bodies of hormone-building blocks.

- Statins and aging

- Low testosterone and cardiac challenges

- Body signs pointing to compromised cardiac health.

- Earlobe message

- Pink nose and rosy cheeks

- Pause For Thought

- Take Home Nuggets

- Pages for personal notes

Why

The Lancet, a highly valued and respected scientific medical Journal in January 2024, reports many countries, including the United Kingdom have continued to experience an apparent excess of deaths long after the peaks associated with Covid-19 pandemic in 2020 and 2021 (lancet January 2024).

The United Kingdom office for national statistics has calculated that there were 7.2% or 44,255 more deaths registered in the United Kingdom in 2022 based on comparison with the five-year average (excluding 2020). This persisted into 2023 with 8.6% or 28,024 more deaths registered in the first six months of the year than expected.

The continuous mortality investigation (CMI) found a similar excess of 28,500 deaths for the same period.

Since July 2020, the office for health improvement and disparities (OHID) has published estimates of excess mortality for England week by week overall and broken down by age, ethnicity, region, and cause. The model finds that in the period from week ending 3rd June 2022 to 30th June 2023, excess deaths for all causes were relatively greatest for 50 - 64-year-olds. (15% higher than expected), compared with 11% higher for 25-49-year-olds and those under 25 years of age and about 9% higher for those over 65 years old.

The age standardised CMI found similar patterns with the largest relative excess deaths for 2022 observed in the young (20-44 age group) and middle age (45 -64-year-olds).

Several causes, including cardiovascular disease show a relative excess greater than that seen in deaths from all causes (9%) over the same period. Cardiovascular disease accounted for 47% for middle-aged adults 50-64 years of age in the 13-month period, the relative excess for almost all causes of death examined was higher than that seen for all ages.

Deaths involving cardio-vascular disease were 33% higher than expected.

Since deaths from cardiovascular related issues account for almost 50% of the increase in the incidence of death, does it make sense to arrest this upward drift?

Surely, if we are able to arrest this increase by helping you protect your heart, we think that our contribution would be palpable; this bite size handbook aims to do precisely that and in so doing allow you to reclaim your health.

The meaning of cardiovascular health

The heart beats about 2.5 billion times over our average lifetime. During this time, millions of litres of blood are pumped to every part of the body. This flow carries with it oxygen, fuel, hormones, other compounds, and many essential cells. Simultaneously, waste products of metabolism are carried away to the excretory organs so they can be taken away from the body. Occasionally, the heart fails because of poor diet, lack of exercise, smoking, infection, a genetic predisposition, and other factors.

A key contributor to poor cardiac health and blood circulation is a condition called atherosclerosis. This is simply described as the accumulation of pockets of cholesterol-rich gunk inside the arteries – channels which carry blood from the heart to tissues for the most part. These pockets, called plaques, limit blood flow through arteries supplying blood to our various organs. If blood supply to the cardiac muscles is occluded, a heart attack results. If the plaque breaks off it can occlude the blood supply to the vessels supplying blood to the cardiac muscles, leading to a heart attack, or if the plaque travels to our brain a stroke would result.

Many people develop some form of cardiovascular disease (a term used to describe diseases affecting the heart and blood vessels) as they get older, it is not inevitable. A healthy lifestyle, or even lifestyle changes and medications, can help reduce the heart-harming trends like high blood pressure and/or high cholesterol before they can create meaningful cardiovascular damage.

We note an almost 70% decline in mortality from cardiovascular disease, coronary heart disease and strokes in the preceding 30 years between 1979 and 2013, and though this is commendable, we are observing an increase in the total number of cardiovascular disease admissions to hospital between 2005 and 2014. It therefore seems that though we are better at managing the condition when it occurs, we are not getting better at preventing the onset in the first place. To reduce the incidence of this disease we have a few suggestions to increase the blood flow through the various vessels.

Suggestion 1: Donate blood. By regularly donating blood, blood flow is improved, and the act of regularly donating blood helps to keep blood thin and so reduce damage to your blood vessels and prevent potential blockage in your vascular channels. In a Finnish study it was found that men who donated blood regularly had an 88% smaller chance of having a heart attack than men who did not donate blood. This may be extrapolated as an explanation for why menstruating women rarely have heart attacks and strokes.

Suggestion 2: Add more garlic to your diet. Garlic, although more widely used for cooking, as an additive to your meal preparation has been found to render blood less sticky. In the blood are some small elements called platelets which are sticky and come together to form a clot to prevent an individual from bleeding out, with trauma, when they work well. By causing blood to be less sticky, it tends to flow better and so reduces the risk of blood clot formation. In some people it has also been shown to lower blood pressure, possibly due to the more laminar blood flow it causes.

Suggestion 3: Add vitamin E as a supplement. Vitamin E is an effective means by which your blood can be thinned. Studies confirm that in over 26 countries, people who had the lowest vitamin E levels had the highest risk of heart disease and stroke. Another study indicated that adding 100 IU of vitamin E a day could reduce your chances of suffering a heart attack by 33%.

Suggestion 4: Omega-3. The omega-3 commonly found in fish oil not only reduces the stickiness of blood, but also reduces inflammation, lowers cholesterol and improves brain health.

With patients on blood-thinning medication caution is advised. We encourage you to speak to your doctor before commencing vitamin E supplements to ensure that the blood-thinning agent you are on does not work synergistically with omega-3 to cause your blood to be too thin.

Suggestion 5: The virtues of water intake continue to be extolled and for good reason. Blood can be thinned by increasing your intake of water. This is particularly important if one has a family history of heart attacks and strokes. It is also advised that you remain well hydrated if you are undertaking any journey involving minimal activity, particularly for journeys exceeding four hours.

Statins and the cholesterol story

It appears that the current aggressiveness with which we aim to lower cholesterol levels may be misguided. Almost without thought, if an individual has a stroke or heart attack, his doctor almost with a sort of knee-jerk reaction prescribes, among other preparations, a cholesterol- lowering drug. This practice, though mainstream, seems to be dangerously fraudulent and engineered by the pharmacological industry.

It seems that our bodies need cholesterol to function. Our brains are mostly made of cholesterol, and many of our hormones are also similarly composed. The very backbone of our major sex hormones, testosterone and oestrogen, are made of cholesterol.

Statins rob our bodies of hormone-building blocks

Aggressively lowering our cholesterol seems to be in direct conflict with our body's need for building blocks. Essentially as our body struggles to increase its hormone levels, we are robbing it of the very building blocks it needs.

Only 10–25% of the cholesterol in our body comes from the foods we eat; 75–90% of our body's cholesterol is made in our livers. This is necessary to enable our bodies to perform major and crucial life functions.

To have sex hormones such as testosterone, progesterone, and oestrogen, as well as the stress hormone cortisol, our body takes cholesterol made in the liver and converts it into pregnenolone. Pregnenolone is then converted into progesterone, which is eventually converted to cortisol, oestrogen, and testosterone along the steroid pathway.

Both low-density lipoprotein (LDL) and total cholesterol levels rise in women as they enter the menopause. A 2009 study in which women were followed for ten years revealed that their total and LDL cholesterol dramatically rose in the year before stopping their periods. Could this spike be the result of a reduced demand for cholesterol downstream, as there is less of a need to produce the female sex hormones of oestrogen and progesterone?

Statins and aging

A woman's cholesterol levels spike at menopause because her ovaries begin to slow down sex hormone production; her body, though, craves more of the hormones. As her levels of oestrogen and progesterone drop, her body starts producing more cholesterol to increase the production of oestrogen and progesterone, so that the impact of aging can be delayed. The introduction of statins, though, causes a competition with the pituitary gland: as it signals the need for more cholesterol or building blocks, the statin freezes the cholesterol production in the liver. This statin therefore induces numerous side effects, including fast-forwarding the aging process in women as a result.

Men do not experience this sharp decline in their hormone production, and as a result their cholesterol levels don't rise as dramatically. However, statins do cause testosterone levels to drop as per a recent European study.

Low testosterone and cardiac challenges

Low testosterone is linked to heart problems: that is, by lowering men's cholesterol artificially with statins, we are likely challenging their heart health as well as accelerating the aging process. Statins therefore rob us of resources our bodies need to create the hormones necessary for keeping our bodies young. Statins are negatively impacting us by keeping us hormone-deficient, with the consequence of us developing weak muscles, mushy memories, and a feeling of old age. In one study 41 patients with high cholesterol were given bioidentical steroid hormones to replace those they had lost during normal aging. It was found that their cholesterol levels fell, and all the patients reported a significant improvement in their quality of life.

Body signs pointing to compromised cardiac health

It is not unusual for the body to give off signs that all is not well; in fact, if we pay attention and listen to our bodies, we will almost always be assured of being able to identify the ailing organ. These signs, though, may not always be accurate, and self-diagnosis is fraught with difficulties.

Earlobe message

Diagonal creases across your earlobes may be a sign of increased susceptibility to cardiovascular disease. If you can identify this marker, a battery of investigations including total cholesterol, triglyceride, homocysteine, and C-reactive protein levels should be checked.

Pink nose and rosy cheeks

Dilated capillaries in your cheeks and nose could be a sign of low stomach acidity. This may indicate that important nutrients, supplements and/or medications are not properly digested and/or absorbed.

Additionally, low production of hydrochloric acid and pepsin in the stomach is associated with hardened arteries, high cholesterol, high triglycerides, high blood pressure and even obesity, all of which are unfriendly to the heart.

Pause For Thought

- Can a poor diet, lack of exercise, smoking, infection and our genes increase our chances of developing cardiovascular disease?
- Can regular donation of blood help to reduce my risk of developing cardiovascular disease?
- Can increased garlic consumption reduce my risk of developing cardiovascular disease?
- Are there any Cardiac benefits to Vitamin E supplements?
- Can omega -3 supplements contribute to my heart health?

- How can drinking water improve my cardiovascular Health?

- Are there any earlobe signs which may tell me about my cardiovascular health?

- Can pink nose and rosy cheeks tell anything about cardiovascular health?

Take Home Nuggets

- One's diet, exercise activity levels, smoking cessation, infections and our genes can all influence our cardiovascular health.

- Regular blood donation, increased garlic consumption, vitamin-E supplements as well as omega-3 supplements and increase water intake are all necessary for ensuring cardiovascular health.

- Ear Lobe appearance, pink nose and rosy cheeks may inform us on our cardiovascular health.

Notes

_____

_____

_____

_____

_____

_____

_____

_____

_____

_____

_____

_____

_____

_____

_____

_____

_____

_____

_____

_____

_____

_____

Notes

_____

_____

_____

_____

_____

_____

_____

_____

_____

_____

_____

_____

_____

_____

_____

_____

_____

_____

_____

_____

_____

_____

_____

Chapter 2
The Cholesterol Confusion

- What is cholesterol?

- Benefits of cholesterol

- Types of cholesterol

- LDL and the pathogenesis of atherosclerotic vascular disease

- How does HDL work?

- Can HDL be oxidised?

- Cholesterol - a more detailed view

- Cholesterol and its usefulness

- LDL v HDL

- Oxidised LDL

- Making use of the test for oxidised LDL

- Steps to drive the oxidised LDL down

- Cholesterol – fighting supplements

- Pause For Thought

- Take Home Nuggets

- Pages for personal notes

Cholesterol is a waxy, fatlike substance in the blood. Much is said about cholesterol, but it is most spoken of as a substance which is bad for your wellbeing. We know that after a cardiac attack and/or stroke, if you survive, the medications you are invariably prescribed by your doctor include a statin to lower your cholesterol levels.

We have learned that 75–90% of our cholesterol is produced by our livers; this then leaves us in a quandary as to why a substance so heavily produced by our bodies is dangerous to our wellbeing. Have we got it wrong? or is it that the body is trying to destroy itself? We see that there is an increase in the levels of cholesterol as a woman enters the menopause, and, though not so dramatically, there is also an increase in cholesterol in the older male. What does that tell us? Could it be that cholesterol is useful to us in our younger years, but as we get older it is no longer needed? Could it be that the cholesterol in our bodies has a definite usefulness, and it is not all bad? If that premise is correct, could it be that the 25% of the available cholesterol that we obtain through our diet is culpable for the bad name given to cholesterol? Our dietary cholesterol comes from the foods we consume, primarily animal/dairy products like meat, eggs, cheese, and milk. Is it the dietary cholesterol which can lead to health problems if it gets too high? Studies suggest an ideal LDL level is at or below 100mg/dL. Or could it be that a potential chemical transformation converts cholesterol to a compound that leads to the ill effects of cholesterol and hence its bad name?

Benefits of cholesterol

As stated in the previous chapter, cholesterol has a significant benefit to human beings in that it serves as a template from which several useful hormones as well as vitamins are synthesised. The value of cholesterol in the synthesis of hormones is supported by the rise in the levels of cholesterol in the body when there is a smaller demand for certain hormones – the sex hormones. We are told that, through the steroid pathway, the body can convert cholesterol into important steroid hormones vital to normal living. Not only this, but a significant portion of our brains is made of cholesterol. This therefore argues for the need for continued cholesterol production by our livers. So, are we saying that cholesterol is both good and bad? If that is the case, how does the body know and why would it utilise its reserve to produce a substance that may be bad for our general wellbeing?

Types of cholesterol

For simplicity, there are two main types of cholesterol, low-density lipoproteins (LDL) or bad cholesterol (which makes up most of your body's cholesterol) and high-density lipoprotein (HDL) or good cholesterol, so called because high levels of HDL cholesterol can reduce the risk of heart disease and strokes by facilitating the excretion of LDL. LDL cholesterol, or low-density lipoprotein cholesterol, is a fat that circulates in the blood, moving cholesterol around the body to the locations where it is needed for cell repair, and it also deposits cholesterol inside of artery walls.

The significance of this is that a high triglyceride level combined with high LDL (bad cholesterol), or low HDL (good cholesterol) is linked with fatty build-ups within the artery walls, which increase the risk of heart attack and strokes.

Interestingly our bodies produce 75-90% of all cholesterol we need. This cholesterol produced by our bodies, in the liver to be exact, is used in the synthesis of cells, certain vitamins and hormones. It therefore seems that our dietary cholesterol should be the point of our focus. Even more precise LDL, particularly the oxidised variety, of which there are two recognised varieties, tend to behave differently. There is the minimally oxidised variety, mmLDL, which is recognised by the LDL receptors, but not by most of the scavenger receptors, and the fully oxidised variety which is recognised by a variety of scavenger receptors but not by the LDL receptor. The biological activity of the mmLDL differs from that of the fully oxidised form. This biological activity includes induction of chemotactic or proinflammatory proteins by endothelial cells and macrophages. It is generally accepted that the oxidation of LDL occurs mostly in the subendothelial space of arteries, and not in the circulation. Small but significant amounts of oxidised LDL (predominantly the mmLDL variety) are immunologically detectable in normal plasma, and the levels are increased in several disease states such as coronary heart disease, diabetes, and renal disease. LDL, therefore, seems to be the template from which the mmLDL variety or the fully oxidised variety is made, so it seems to be the primary culprit in the genesis of vascular disease, hence its sobriquet 'bad cholesterol'.

LDL and the pathogenesis of atherosclerotic vascular disease

There are many lines of evidence which suggest that oxidised low-density lipoprotein is implicated in the pathogenesis of atherosclerotic vascular disease.

LDL oxidation seems to be catalysed by transition metal ions, and several free radicals, as well as some oxidising enzymes. LDL oxidation is an early event in atherosclerosis, and oxidised LDL contributes to atherogenesis. This is evidenced by the development of foam cells in vitro and the presence of oxidised LDL in vivo. Oxidised LDL has a number of proatherogenic potentials such as stimulation of endothelial cells and monocytes towards increased inflammatory cytokines, chemokines and adhesion molecules, stimulations of macrocytes/macrophages towards the increased tissue factor, matrix metalloproteinase and scavenger receptors, eventually leading to foam cell formation of macrophages and the progression of atherosclerotic lesions. It is believed that LDL oxidation does not take place in the circulation and must occur in the arterial wall because serum lipoprotein lipids are well protected from oxidation by the robust antioxidant defences, and LDL itself contains mostly alpha tocopherol, an antioxidant vitamin, as a major transport vehicle.

The above paragraph, though difficult to read, can be simply summarised by indicating that oxidised LDL induces atherosclerosis (a condition in which your arteries are narrowed, making it difficult for blood to flow through them). This increases the risk of heart attack and strokes.

It therefore seems the LDL is atherosclerotic, only on its conversion into its oxidised form.

How does HDL work?

HDL cholesterol absorbs LDL cholesterol in the blood and carries it back to the liver. The liver then flushes it from the body. High levels of HDL cholesterol can lower your risk of heart disease and stroke, but can the levels of HDL be too high? Individuals with very high HDL cholesterol levels above 60mg/dL were nearly 50% more likely to have a heart attack or die from heart disease than people whose HDL levels were 41–60mg/dL. HDL can reduce ischaemia/reperfusion injury by inhibiting damaging processes and by protective responses elicited by tissue after ischaemia/reperfusion. HDL exert their effect on different cell types, as cardiomyocytes, endothelial cells and leukocytes. HDL cholesterol helps rid the body of LDL, or bad cholesterol, and keeps it from collecting on the linings of your arteries. HDL cholesterol appears to make individuals less susceptible to the development of atherosclerosis. HDL appears to have three important roles in the body. Its main function is to efflux cholesterol and other lipids from peripheral tissues (such as the cardiovascular system) and transport them to either (a) the liver for disposal, or (b) steroidogenic tissue to support hormone production; or (c) to exchange lipids with apoB-containing particles (apoB particles are the basic unit of injury to the arterial wall).

Can HDL cholesterol be oxidised?

Since HDL has the basic cholesterol structure, it can be oxidised; but in its oxidised form it seems to behave very differently from the oxidised LDL. Whereas oxidised LDL is atherosclerotic and contributes to atherogenesis, when HDL is oxidised, it is believed to have a pivotal role in the onset and progression of atherosclerotic plaque. It may therefore serve as a pointer to the presence of atherosclerosis and cardiovascular disease.

Cholesterol – a more detailed view

Much has been said about cholesterol and its impact on heart disease. We have been told about good cholesterol (HDL) and bad cholesterol (LDL). We place patients on cholesterol-lowering drugs called statins which theoretically should increase our levels of good cholesterol and reduce our levels of bad cholesterol. Unfortunately, even while taking these statins patients continue to die with cardiac events, which doubtlessly raises the question: Do statins do what is said on the tin? Or are we unclear as to the way cholesterol produces its anticardiac effect?

Cholesterol and its usefulness

Cholesterol is subdivided into two types: (a) high-density lipoprotein cholesterol (HDL), or good cholesterol; and (b) and low-density lipoprotein cholesterol (LDL), or bad cholesterol.

Much of what is written about cholesterol highlights the ill effect of LDL, and there is only a cursory mention of its preferred relative, HDL. We know that 75% to 90% of the cholesterol needed by the body is produced by the liver. It would therefore seem that cholesterol is needed in the body and plays a meaningful role. We talk of cholesterol involvement in the synthesis of several hormones, notably the steroid or sex hormones and the stress hormones. It is also involved in the synthesis of vitamins and forms an integral component of the cell membrane.

LDL v HDL

LDL is called bad cholesterol because high levels of LDL lead to a build-up of cholesterol in one's arteries, but not only that: LDL cholesterol is also involved in transporting antioxidants, building muscles and fighting infection. Recognising both the structural and functional role played by cholesterol in the membranes of cells, the transport of cholesterol to the arterial walls is valuable.

HDL is considered good cholesterol because it absorbs cholesterol in the blood and carries it back to the liver. The liver then flushes it from the body. High normal levels of HDL can lower your risk of heart disease and stroke.

If we claim that HDL is the good cholesterol because it absorbs cholesterol in the blood and carries it back to the liver which then flushes it from the body, and we also claim that LDL plays a valuable role in the walls of the arteries, the question is why is cholesterol given a bad name and why are we given toxic substances like statins to reduce its level?

The bad name given to cholesterol is in relation to the cardiovascular system, particularly its effect on the arterial walls. So, what causes a substance which is reputedly good for cell membranes, an integral part of the arterial walls, to be bad?

Oxidised LDL

LDL molecules in our arterial walls become damaged by oxygen molecules, a process called oxidation. This is very similar to the effect one observes when metallic tools are left exposed to the elements, specifically water and oxygen. These metal objects undergo oxidation and corrode, leading to the weakening of the metal. This is what happens with LDL cholesterol, and it is in this state that it becomes deadly to humans.

Oxidised LDL-cholesterol attracts the type of inflammatory immune cells called macrophages. These macrophages start devouring these oxidised LDL particles in the arterial walls. These macrophages, after eating up these oxidised LDL particles, become transformed into fat-laden foam cells which cause more inflammation in the artery walls.

In addition to this inflammatory process, the oxidised LDL cholesterol encourages the formation of arterial plaque, the result of which is a progressive narrowing of your arteries. That is not all, though: the plaques may rupture, and bits may enter the circulation, leading to a heart attack or even a stroke, both of which can be deadly. So not only is oxidised LDL atherosclerotic (causing narrowing of the blood vessels), it also makes them inelastic, it encourages plaque formation and can rupture with deadly consequences. Hence the rationale for considering oxidised LDL cholesterol as bad. LDL is useful until it becomes oxidised. Unfortunately, our General Practitioners, our primary health care doctors, do not routinely screen for oxidised LDL levels which would be a more useful indicator of cardiovascular risk than routine screening for LDL, HDL and triglycerides. Mainstream medicine has failed to do the right investigations and their approach to treatment does not seem to be evidence-based. A huge meta-analysis of 65,000 people published in Evidence-Based Medicine found no link between statin drugs and living longer. In fact, researchers did not find any relationship between cholesterol levels and survival rates. These findings must be taken in conjunction with the known side effects of statins, including increased risk of cancer, muscle damage, liver damage, kidney damage and memory loss.

Making use of the test for oxidised LDL

Using the available test for oxidised LDL must be addressed if we are to have greater success against the scourge of oxidised LDL. Hopefully with time this test for oxidised LDL will become more widely available.

Research clearly shows that oxidised LDL levels are linked to heart disease, and it serves as a useful warning sign for future heart attacks and strokes. In a study published in the journal Circulation, the plasma oxidised LDL levels rose sharply above 3.5-fold in patients who have had a heart attack or stroke over control subjects who had no such event.

Studies have revealed that the best marker to distinguish between people with and without coronary artery disease is the ratio of oxidised LDL to HDL cholesterol. This ratio is a far better predictor of heart disease than the standard total cholesterol or LDL cholesterol measurements.

With the more widespread utilisation of the test to measure oxidised LDL levels, we also need to change our focus. We need to determine how best to keep oxidised LDL levels low. While developing methods, before we can do this, we need to understand what triggers the oxidation of LDL.

Steps to drive the oxidised LDL down

We can start with our diets. Several studies have shown that Mediterranean-style diets, diets of plant-based foods such as whole grains, vegetables, legumes, fruits, nuts, seeds, herbs and spices, reduce LDL oxidation. A study of 372 adults at high risk of heart disease found that diets rich in olive oil and nuts caused oxidised LDL levels to drop. In contrast, people following low-fat diets had no change in their oxidised LDL levels. Diets rich in polyunsaturated fats like those in fast foods, junk foods and baked goods increased the oxidised LDL levels. In fact, corn oil, sunflower oil, safflower oil, cottonseed oil and soy oil all seem to raise oxidised LDL levels. Both vegan and gluten-free diets have been shown to reduce oxidised LDL levels. Flavonoids in pomegranate juice have been shown to protect against oxidation of LDL. Green tea also fights against LDL oxidation.

Cholesterol-fighting supplements

Vitamin E is a powerful antioxidant that destroys free radicals and prevents oxidation damage in the body. Food sources of vitamin E include brown rice, seeds and nuts. The supplement coenzyme Q10 targets and reduces the oxidation of LDL cholesterol. This substance can be obtained from seafood, peanuts, and meat, or can be acquired online in capsule form which you can take at a dose of 60–200mg per day. Garlic and grape seed extract are also thought to be useful in protecting against the formation of oxidised LDL.

Unfortunately, hormonal imbalance can facilitate oxidation of LDL. In this case the thyroid gland is a major culprit: both hypothyroidism and hyperthyroidism increase the oxidation of LDL cholesterol. It is also likely that oestrogen can fight

LDL oxidation. Chronic infections are yet another factor that increases your oxidised LDL levels.

In this regard, it would be advisable to consume foods that will tend to decrease the likelihood of promoting oxidised LDL while simultaneously you check your hormonal levels, ensuring that any imbalance is corrected.

Pause For Thought

- Do our bodies produce cholesterol?
- What are the major types of cholesterol?
- If our bodies produce cholesterol, why is it given a bad name?
- Are there any benefits to cholesterol in our bodies?
- Are there any ill effects to cholesterol?
- How does good cholesterol work?
- Can we identify oxidised LDL cholesterol?
- Can we decrease levels of oxidised LDL in our bodies?

Take Home Nuggets

- Our body produces about 75% to 90% of all the cholesterol it needs. This is mainly produced in our livers by an enzyme called HMG-Co-A.
- The two major types of cholesterol in our bodies are HDL (high Density Lipoprotein cholesterol) and LDL (low density lipoprotein cholesterol).

- Cholesterol has important uses in the body, it is involved in the structure of cell membranes, production of certain hormones and in the production of vitamin D.

- The LDL which is produced in larger quantities and is of greater utility in the body can be deposited in the walls of our blood vessels where it becomes oxidised and it is this oxidised variety which is harmful to the cardiovascular system.

- HDL on the other hand is considered good cholesterol because it helps the body reduce its LdL load by transporting it to sites where it can be excreted from the body.

- There are available blood tests which can be done to predict the presence of oxidised LDL and we can also reduce our levels of oxidised LDL in our bodies.

Notes

Notes

_____

_____

_____

_____

_____

_____

_____

_____

_____

_____

_____

_____

_____

_____

_____

_____

_____

_____

_____

_____

Chapter 3
Lowering Your LDL Cholesterol

- Commonly used steps to lower one's LDL cholesterol

- The role of statins

- Addressing atherosclerosis without statins

- Approaches to cholesterol-lowering diets

- Red yeast rice

- Pause For Thought

- Take Home Nuggets

- Pages for personal notes

Since our research to date reveals that LDL is the bad cholesterol and oxidation of this cholesterol triggers an inflammatory response and simultaneously is also atherosclerotic, a sensible approach to avoiding this deadly toll on heart health can be addressed from at least four pathways. Firstly, one can attempt to reduce or avoid the intake of known cholesterol- containing foods. Secondly, one can move to increase the amount of HDL cholesterol (the good cholesterol) to which our bodies become exposed. Thirdly, trying to ensure that the LDL remains in circulation in the vascular system and not deposited in the walls of the vascular system. And fourthly, one can try to keep the LDL cholesterol deposited in the walls of the vascular system free from oxidation.

With these approaches, one would expect some success in addressing cardiovascular disease. There are five different statins available on prescription in the UK, and seven available in the USA, each generation of statin claiming to be superior to the previous generation. The flippant among us will claim that when there are several preparations designed to do the same task, none is good at the task, and that may explain why there is an effort to continue to produce other substances hoping that they are superior to their predecessors. I leave you to draw your own conclusions.

The role of statins

Statins decrease your LDL or bad cholesterol and may increase your HDL or good cholesterol. HDL increase is desirable, since it helps the body to get rid of LDL cholesterol. Statins are believed to work by interfering with the liver's ability to produce cholesterol. They block the enzyme necessary for the liver to make cholesterol. Seeing that 75–90% of the body's cholesterol is made in the liver, shutting down that process will impact on the cholesterol-dependent processes in our bodies, leading to a raft of side effects which may be unpleasant. We obtain only 10–25% of our body's cholesterol needs from the foods we eat. So, although statins can lower the levels of LDL, based on the known mechanism by which it brings about its effects, it would seem to have a negligible effect on dietary LDL. However, statins are claimed to be able to lower the levels of LDL in the blood. Statins, by their prescribed modality of function, address two of the four approaches listed above, but patients on statins tend to experience significant side effects, not least a drop in vital hormones, like testosterone and the stress hormone, cortisol. Other known side effects include headaches, dizziness, nausea, fatigue and unusual weakness, digestive system problems such as constipation, diarrhoea, indigestion and flatulence, muscle pains, sleep problems and thrombocytopaenia. In a recent report a 47-year-old man from Wales claimed that he is unable to walk and is wheelchair-bound after using a statin for four years. The report states that he had fevers, muscle aches and high temperatures at night, and over nine months he lost his ability to walk. He has since been diagnosed with necrotising myopathy, a rare autoimmune condition which causes chronic loss of muscle. tissue and weakness. He has said he had no problems until, commencing use of the statin, he found himself struggling to get out of bed. He is now unable to walk and is wheelchair- bound. As part of his care, he was advised to stop taking the statins.

With these side effects, the number of statins on the market, and their apparent failure in bringing about the desired effects, despite claims that they effectively lower bad cholesterol and increase good cholesterol, people on statins continue to die with coronary vascular disease; it seems that (a) statins are not the ideal preparation for treating and addressing cardiovascular disease even after a cardiovascular event; or (b) we may not have understood the mechanism by which cholesterol impacts the cardiovascular system.

Addressing atherosclerosis without statins

There are means by which one can drop one's cholesterol levels significantly without the use of statins. The generally held view is that saturated fats are bad and unsaturated fats are good, but the Atkins Diet, which promotes high fats and high proteins in your diet, has led us to realise that the process is not as simple. We contend that only man-made fats should always be avoided, particularly hydrogenated and partially hydrogenated vegetable oils. These oils are almost ubiquitous and present in a lot of food commonly used as snacks. The best food sources for fatty acids are fish and unroasted nuts and seeds.

Several vitamins, minerals and botanicals are known to lower cholesterol. Some of these include inositol hexaniacinate, lecithin, pantethine, L-carnitine, beta-sitosterol, fish oil, phosphatidylcholine, choline, vitamin C, calcium, vanadium, magnesium, chromium, and vitamin E. All these compounds do exactly what statins are supposed to do but without the horrible side effects listed above.

There are also botanicals, including guggulipid, garlic oil, red yeast rice, ginger, pectin, curcumin, fenugreek powder, reishi mushrooms, silymarin, turmeric, Garcinia, and artichokes which behave in a similar manner to statins but without the side effects. Sugar cane provides a natural supplement called policosanol, which may be the most effective way to lower your cholesterol naturally. This compound has been shown to be more effective in lowering bad cholesterol than statins, and it also lowers triglycerides and elevates HDL levels. It does not require a prescription and is even available online. As an additional benefit there are none of the side effects seen when statins are used.

Although much of the discussion hovers around high cholesterol and its association with heart disease, low cholesterol carries a risk of cancer, stroke, and depression. Cholesterol is an essential building block for steroid hormones such as dehydroepiandrosterone (DHEA), oestrogens, progesterone and pregnenolone. It is also a key component of every cell membrane in our body. So we must aim for a cholesterol level in the blood within a certain range. A high serum cholesterol is usually considered to have a value above 200mg/dL, whereas a low cholesterol refers to a value at or below 160.

Approaches to cholesterol-lowering diets

There are two basic approaches to cholesterol-lowering diets, both of which can work. Approach 1: A low-fat, high-complex carbohydrate plan. Approach 2: The high-protein, low-carbohydrate approach. High-protein diets work well for many people struggling with cholesterol problems because these individuals' bodies generally manufacture much more insulin than others in response to refined sugar and excess carbs. This overproduction of insulin causes the liver to produce too much total cholesterol and triglycerides, and not enough HDL. Some people have a predisposition to high increase in insulin levels in response to sugar and carbohydrate intake; this causes the insulin to not work properly and fails to take the sugar into the cells of the body: this is interpreted as having insufficient insulin and so the body produces more insulin. This excess insulin is associated with the onset of high blood pressure and cholesterol anomalies.

Carbohydrates and saturated fats get a bad name for causing high levels of cholesterol, but they account for just about 50% of cases of high cholesterol. It therefore seems that factors other than your diet are responsible for the other cases of high serum cholesterol. Japanese researchers have found that small quantities of lead caused elevated levels of cholesterol in animal studies. Lead appears to be able to do this in two ways: (1) it induces the gene responsible for creating the liver enzymes that produce cholesterol; and (2) it also suppresses the production of liver enzymes necessary for the breakdown and destruction of cholesterol.

Red yeast rice

Red yeast rice is a bright reddish-purple fermented rice, which acquires its colour from being cultivated with mould Monascus purpureus. In a study published in Annals of Internal Medicine involving 62 patients who had stopped taking statins because of terrible pains, were placed in two groups. One group was given 3 600mg capsules of red yeast rice or placebo two times a day for 26 weeks. Both groups also made lifestyle changes, incorporating diet and exercise plans, yoga, and massage.

The red yeast rice worked, bringing on a 35-point drop in LDL cholesterol. The group placed on placebo but who also made lifestyle changes saw only a 15-point drop. There were no unwanted side effects in this study, and the results were encouraging.

Pause For Thought

- If we produce 90% of the cholesterol in our bodies, why should we reduce the amount of cholesterol produced?

- There are five different types of Statins licenced for use in the UK and seven different types licensed for use in the USA, why so many?

- What do Statins do?

- Do they have any side effects?

- Are there any other options available for lowering cholesterol?

- Does diet have any significant impact on the amount of cholesterol in our bodies?

- Does lead have any impact on the amount of cholesterol in our bodies?

Take Home Nuggets

- If up to 90% of the cholesterol in our bodies is self-produced, why bother about trying to lower the amounts of cholesterol in our body? Science tells us that a form of cholesterol called oxidised LDL cholesterol is harmful to our cardiovascular system. Hence the use of statins to try to lower the amount of cholesterol in our bodies. Statins are believed to produce their effects by inhibiting the activity of the enzyme which produces cholesterol in our bodies but they are associated with numerous side effects. Statins have no impact on a cholesterol rich diet since they work by inhibiting the body's ability to produce cholesterol. Other seemingly unrelated substances such as lead can increase the cholesterol levels in our bodies in at least two separate ways.

Notes

_____

_____

_____

_____

_____

_____

_____

_____

_____

_____

_____

_____

_____

_____

_____

_____

_____

_____

_____

_____

Notes

_____

_____

_____

_____

_____

_____

_____

_____

_____

_____

_____

_____

_____

_____

_____

_____

_____

_____

_____

_____

_____

_____

_____

Chapter 4
Protecting the Heart

- Two common culprits

- Diabetes and heart health

- High blood pressure and heart health

- The effect of cardiotoxins

- Maintaining heart health

- Pomegranate juice

- The role of minerals

- Copper

- Potassium

- Magnesium

- Magnesium and cholesterol balance

- Heart disease and magnesium

- The miracle molecule

- How does it work?

- Pause For Thought

- Take Home Nuggets

- Pages for personal notes

The heart continues to pump from our birth to the time of our death: every effort should be made to keep it as healthy as possible to allow it to work efficiently. We have seen above how oxidised cholesterol can interfere with this process, but are there other factors which can directly or indirectly negatively affect heart health?

We know that chronic ailments like diabetes and hypertension (high blood pressure) can negatively affect heart health, albeit through different mechanisms; we also know that certain substances to which we are exposed can be cardiotoxic, and there are certain steps which we can take to improve our heart health.

Diabetes and heart health

Diabetes is a metabolic disorder that can affect the heart muscles, causing them to contract less efficiently, and it can also negatively affect the diameter of the arteries through which the blood is pumped. As stated above, the blood vessels are narrowed through the impact of excessive insulin on the cholesterol, producing and destroying enzymes in the liver. Simply put, diabetes is toxic to the heart. It reduces the diameter of the blood vessels, causing the heart to generate a greater force to push the blood around our bodies, whilst simultaneously causing the muscles of the heart walls to contract less efficiently, a recipe for heart failure. Minimising the effect of diabetes on the heart is best done by not ever developing diabetes. If one has been diagnosed with diabetes, however, the impact of this deadly disease on the heart can be minimised by the effective control of the disease process. The effective control and defeat of this disease are beyond the scope of this book. It is, however, covered in clear detail in the book in this series, Defeating Diabetes.

High blood pressure and heart health

This is a major risk factor for heart disease. It is the result of the pressure of the blood in your arteries and other vessels being too high. This high blood pressure, if not controlled, can affect the heart. The way it is believed to damage the vascular system is through the damage in the arterial wall which leads to scarring and reduction in the elasticity of these blood vessels. The result is increased blood pressure and decreased supply of blood to the various organs, the heart included, thus leading to heart disease. The decreased blood flow is believed to be caused, in part, by the oxidation of low-density lipoprotein (LDL) – the bad cholesterol and the atherosclerotic potential of this oxidised compound. More on the way high blood pressure leads to heart disease and how best to manage this condition will be addressed later in this book.

The effect of cardiotoxins

Our bodies are repeatedly exposed to a variety of substances, some of which are toxic to the heart. The term cardiotoxins is usually reserved for anti-cancer chemical agents that are known to damage the heart. These Cardiotoxic agents include alkylating agents like cyclophosphamide, ifosfamide, cisplatin, busulfan and mitomycin. Other classes of anti-cancer drugs known as angiogenesis inhibitors, which include thalidomide, lenalidomide and pomalidomide are also toxic to the heart. Still a third class of drugs known as anthracycline agents are toxic to the heart. These include doxorubicin, daunorubicin, epirubicin, idarubicin and mitoxantrone. However, there are other agents which are toxic to the heart, even some socially tolerated preparations that are known to be damaging either directly or indirectly to the heart. We talk of alcohol, cigarette smoke and hard drugs like cocaine etc.

Alkylating agents are believed to cause damage to the heart by destroying cardiac cells. The damage is therefore irreversible.

Angiogenesis inhibitors are believed to increase the risk of hypertension, arterial thromboembolism, cardiac ischaemia, and cardiac dysfunction.

Anthracycline agent-induced cardiotoxicity is due to the generation of free radicals which destroy heart cells, thereby weakening cardiac muscles leading to left ventricular dysfunction and congestive heart failure.

Maintaining heart health

Dental problems can impact on heart health. Researchers from University College London found that people who brush their teeth less than twice per day had up to a 70% risk of heart disease. This is strongly suggestive that you should aim to brush your teeth at least twice per day.

Pomegranate juice

This juice, which is widely available in many health food stores and supermarkets, contains a blend of powerful disease-fighting antioxidants which include phenolic compounds, tannins, and anthocyanins.

Norwegian researchers have found that pomegranates contain a higher concentration of antioxidants than 23 other fruits. It has 10 times more antioxidants than grapes, oranges, plums, pineapples, lemons, dates, clementines and grapefruit.

One of its major benefits is that it prevents the oxidation of LDL, a major cause of arterial damage and plaque build-up.

Israeli researchers have found that this juice reduces LDL oxidation by some 40%. It has also been shown to reduce the build-up of plaque in the carotid or neck arteries which supply the brain. It is particularly helpful for people with diabetes: it leads to a significant reduction in both total cholesterol and LDL cholesterol levels.

The role of minerals

Copper

The standard advice from the establishment on how best to protect your heart is to lose weight, stay away from fattening foods, and embark on an exercise programme. Whilst this is excellent advice, many still succumb to heart disease even at a very young age. One therefore wonders: is there any other approach which can be used in conjunction with the above advice to maintain heart health?

Copper plays an important role in many enzyme reactions and is involved in bone and connective tissue construction. It also helps to prevent oxidation of fatty acids that can destroy both DNA and cell membranes. It is involved in absorbing, utilising and synthesising the oxygen carrier, haemoglobin. Furthermore, copper helps to maintain the integrity of the myelin which covers nerves, keeping them protected from injury and deterioration. Most of the copper in our bodies is found in the liver where it contributes to energy and detoxification mechanisms. So how is copper involved in heart health? I hear you ask.

Too little copper is associated with high cholesterol, high blood pressure and irregular heart rhythms, including atrial fibrillation. In proper balance with zinc, copper acts as an antioxidant, removes free radicals and protects the heart.

Atrial fibrillation is a condition of the heart that causes an irregular and often abnormally fast heart rate. A regular heart rate should beat between 60 and 100 times a minute. Atrial fibrillation is associated with symptoms and a risk of stroke.

Shockingly, up to 33% of the population may not have enough copper in their diet. In the presence of atrial fibrillation, it has been found that there is a higher zinc/copper ratio in the diets of the affected individuals. It means that the correct balance of both minerals is necessary. A high ratio of zinc to copper, rather than copper to zinc, can cause heart problems.

It has been found that copper can help solve atrial fibrillation as well as premature ventricular contractions.

Taking 4mg of copper each day significantly reduces or extinguishes premature ventricular contractions. The recommended daily amount of copper is 1.5–3mg. This can be had through the consumption of meat, shellfish, legumes, Brazil nuts and cashews.

Potassium

If your potassium levels are too high, this will have a negative impact on cardiac function; similarly, if too low the same is likely to occur. Potassium is critical for our nerves and heart. A study published in the Journal of the American Medical Association (JAMA), *Internal Medicine*, with data from the National Health and Nutrition Examination Survey, found that people in the upper-quartile range for potassium were less likely to die or suffer heart attacks or strokes. So, what constitutes the lower and upper quartiles? In the NHANES study, the lowest quartile of potassium intake was about 1.8g a day, and in the highest quartile the intake was about 4g per day.

The mortality benefits with higher intake are very significant, up to a third less. How we increase our potassium intake could be through our diet or with supplements.

Potassium supplements are not recommended since they are allowed to have a maximum of only 99mg of potassium. The typical Western diet of refined grains, sugars and refined vegetables is low in potassium. Root vegetables like beets, carrots and Turnips are a very good source of potassium. Vegetable sources such as spinach and kale can provide up to 2.5 g/pound. Bananas are also a good source of potassium, but which I will not recommend because they also expose you to sugar, particularly fructose, which may not be healthy if you suffer from specific chronic ailments.

Magnesium

You may have been exposed to supplemental magnesium from childhood in the form of Epsom Salts, which were used by our parents for a variety of purposes. This mineral helps to promote everything from strong bones to a good night's sleep. There is now a growing body of research suggesting that magnesium can hold the key to protecting your heart, and even stopping a deadly attack before it strikes.

Inflammation is the hidden culprit which starts breaking down our bodies and eventually leads to chronic diseases, including that of the cardiovascular system. This process is believed to commence when the cells lining the vascular channels, the endothelium, become inflamed. This inflammation triggers the body's inflammatory response with the production of C-reactive proteins, nuclear factor kappa B, and cytokines and platelets are also brought to the area. The body attempts to heal this area with a patch made of cholesterol, platelets and other factors. This patch later collects calcium and fibrous tissue and hardens into a plaque which obstructs blood flow through the arteries, leading to a condition called atherosclerosis.

Research is now indicating that with adequate amounts of magnesium, this inflammatory response is less likely to occur. In one study rabbits with varying levels of cholesterol were fed diets with varying levels of magnesium. The findings were that rabbits with high levels of cholesterol, but low levels of magnesium developed significant atherosclerosis, but in those with high levels of cholesterol and being on a diet with high levels of magnesium, these rabbits were almost plaque-free. Dietary magnesium based on this, and several other studies has been advanced as being able to prevent arterial plaque formation and therefore prevent atherosclerotic cardiovascular disease.

Additionally, magnesium can block calcium channels and so prevent too much muscle contraction. This is applicable not only to peripheral muscle groups, but also to heart muscle, keeping the heart muscle sufficiently relaxed and preventing a heart attack.

Magnesium and cholesterol balance

Magnesium helps to maintain cholesterol balance. Its presence is necessary for the normal functioning of many enzymes, including lipoprotein lipase, the enzyme which increases the level of good cholesterol (HDL) while it keeps triglycerides from getting too high.

Through its role in the metabolism of lecithin, magnesium is also able to lower the bad cholesterol, LDL.

Magnesium is also able to work through the same pathway as statins by inhibiting HMG-CoA, the enzyme that makes cholesterol in our bodies without the same side effect profile and risks that are caused by statins.

Heart disease and magnesium

Even in the presence of atherosclerotic cardiovascular disease (ASCVD), studies show that magnesium can prevent it from getting any worse and can even lead to an improvement of your condition. The severity of ASCVD is usually judged by measuring the carotid intima-media thickness (CIMT): the thicker the artery, the more severe the condition. In a study in which patients were given 100mg of magnesium daily for two months, there was a reduction in these patients' CIMT. The reverse is also true: the Atherosclerosis Risk in Communities (ARIC) study showed that low levels of magnesium intake resulted in thicker arteries. This was more significant in women than in men. Other studies have also confirmed that women are more susceptible to cardiovascular damage associated with low magnesium intake.

In a study of 240,000 patients treated with 100mg of magnesium daily, there was an 8% reduction in strokes resulting from arterial blockage. Risk of strokes is also increased by atrial fibrillation, a complication of cardiovascular surgery which is lessened by preoperative magnesium sulphate infusion. The incidence of this complication in two similar groups revealed that the incidence in the untreated group was 21%, whilst in the treated group there was only a 2% incidence.

The miracle molecule

We have spoken ad nauseam about the underlying impact of narrowing vasculature on cardiovascular disease. In a nutshell, as our blood vessels become increasingly narrower, the work done by the heart is increased, and there is more damage to blood vessels with as if joining a slippery slope. Blood vessels are narrowed, and the heart is forced to work harder as it squeezes blood against the increased resistance.

It is here that this miracle molecule can exert its effect, stop cardiac pains, and reduce the risk of heart attack, stroke and even pull you back from the brink of death from cardiovascular disease. With this miracle molecule, if in short supply, you will be at increased risk of coronary heart disease, heart attack, stroke, diabetes, and Alzheimer's disease, to name a few conditions that are influenced by this miracle molecule.

This molecule, nitric oxide, was named the miracle molecule of the year in 1992. These are some of the effects of this miracle molecule on your overall health:

- It stops artery-clogging blood clots from forming.
- It reverses arterial plaque build-up.
- It prevents high blood pressure.
- It lowers C-reactive protein.
- It reduces the level of triglycerides.

With that Nitric Oxide reduces your risk of heart attack and stroke, two of the major killers of modern times. Additionally, nitric oxide reduces the devastating complications of diabetes, such as kidney disease, blindness, and amputation.

How does it work?

Every cell in our body sends or receives messages through nitric oxide. The most important work of nitric oxide appears to be in the circulatory system. The focus is at the level of the endothelium, which lines every blood vessel in your body. This is where nitric oxide is produced. This nitric oxide enters the smooth muscles of our arteries and signals them to relax. The result is that the vessels dilate, allowing blood flow to increase and flow more easily, with less resistance, so that the cells, tissues, and organs can obtain their full supply of oxygen and nutrients.

Pause For Thought

Can diabetes and high blood pressure impact heart health?

- Are there known cardiotoxic agents?
- Does teeth brushing contribute to heart health?
- Can pomegranate juice contribute to heart health?
- Are there any known minerals which can affect heart health?
- Why is nitric oxide considered a miracle molecule?

Take Home Nuggets

- Both diabetes and high blood pressure affects cardiovascular health, but through different mechanisms.
- Several agents used in medicine are known to be toxic to the heart, among them are a variety of agents used as chemotherapeutic agents in the treatment of cancer.
- Research shows that by brushing your teeth less than twice a day significantly impacts on your cardiac health. It is believed that pomegranate juice makes several positive contributions to heart health.

- There are some minerals for example copper and potassium that can have a negative impact on cardiac health, while others for example magnesium and calcium have a positive impact on cardiac health.

- Nitric oxide has a positive impact on cardiovascular health and is considered a miracle molecule mainly through its ability to dilate blood vessels.

Notes

Notes

_____

_____

_____

_____

_____

_____

_____

_____

_____

_____

_____

_____

_____

_____

_____

_____

_____

_____

_____

_____

_____

Chapter 5
The Broken Heart Syndrome Also Called Takotsubo Cardiomyopathy

- Stress and the heart
- Takotsubo cardiomyopathy
- Diagnosing takotsubo and its natural treatment
- Pause For Thought
- Take home nuggets
- Pages for personal notes

As we tread through life, experiencing a broken heart is almost inevitable, be it at the termination of your first love affair, the loss of a parent, other significant family member or a dear friend. Whatever the cause, we tend to speak of a broken heart figuratively, though there is truly an organic entity called the broken heart syndrome. This entity is sufficiently well known that it is referred to in medical parlance as takotsubo cardiomyopathy. This entity presents like a heart attack, but investigations will reveal that there is no arterial blockage.

This condition can be precipitated by a stressful, sad, or emotionally taxing event. It causes the muscular part of the heart to swell for a period and then break.

It is a medical condition called takotsubo cardiomyopathy, also called "the broken heart syndrome". The heart muscle is stunned by some tragic event and is not able to beat properly and effectively. After 31 years of clinical practice, I have only knowingly met one such patient.

The affected heart has the appearance of a fish pot because the top left side of the heart contracts differently from the bottom part, hence its name. Takotsubo is the Japanese name for a fishing pot used for trapping octopus.

Takotsubo cardiomyopathy

The symptoms include chest pains, shortness of breath, sweating, irregular heartbeat, nausea, fatigue, and vomiting. It is a serious, life-threatening health condition. This syndrome is becoming increasingly recognisable, a case in point being that there were only 315 cases in 2006, but in 2012 the numbers had ballooned to 6,230. It can be picked up both on blood test and on an electrocardiogram (ECG).

Modern medicine is limited in what is available to prevent the occurrence of this condition or to prevent a recurrence.

The bulk of the diagnosed patients do not have the classic risk factors we associate with heart disease – for example, diabetes, high blood pressure, obesity, high cholesterol, or smoking – and interestingly about 90% of these patients are postmenopausal women. The one common factor is that these women are usually anxious and have a high proportion of circulating adrenaline in their blood.

A report in The New England Journal of Medicine has revealed that antihypertension medicines have no effect on the prevention of the recurrence of this condition: the recommendation is for the patient to reduce her levels of stress and anxiety.

Diagnosing takotsubo and its natural treatment

Let us call this patient Agnes (not her real name).

Agnes, a 58-year-old woman, was involved in a horrific car accident which was fatal to three of her colleagues. By the time the road traffic wardens and the ambulance arrived on the scene, she started complaining of chest pains and difficulty breathing. She was rushed to the emergency room.

Blood test and an ECG confirmed that she had a heart attack, but a coronary angiogram was clear, showing no evidence of blockage. She was therefore diagnosed with takotsubo.

On follow-up her cardiologist prescribed some basic medications and advised her that the only way she could avoid a recurrence was to reduce her stress and anxiety levels. This, though, is easier said than done, and he sent the patient to see a psychiatrist.

Agnes, though, had difficulty tolerating antidepressant and anxiolytic medications, so she visited a naturalist. She was placed on magnesium and coenzyme Q10, as well as ribose. With this regime it was hoped that her broken heart could be repaired and simultaneously strengthened so that there would be a smaller chance of a recurrence. Acupuncture sessions and meditation were also recommended to reduce her anxiety levels.

Pause For Thought

- Is there a condition called the broken heart Syndrome?
- Are the number of these cases increasing?
- Is the occurrence of this condition influenced by antihypertensives?
- Can this condition recur?
- Can this condition result from stress?
- Does blood studies and ECG confirm the presence of a heart attack?
- What is the result of a coronary angiogram in this condition?
- Is any blockage of cardiac vessels found on coronary angiogram?

Take Home Nuggets

- This entity, the broken heart syndrome, is real. It usually occurs after a stressful event and mimics a heart attack which is confirmed by blood studies as well as an ECG. However, a coronary angiogram reveals no blockage. It can recur, and its recurrence is unaffected by antihypertensive medications. In this condition the rhythmical beat of the heart is lost and becomes disjointed.

Notes

_____

_____

_____

_____

_____

_____

_____

_____

_____

_____

_____

_____

_____

_____

_____

_____

_____

_____

_____

_____

_____

_____

_____

Notes

_____

_____

_____

_____

_____

_____

_____

_____

_____

_____

_____

_____

_____

_____

_____

_____

_____

_____

_____

_____

Chapter 6
Multifactorial Causes of Heart Disease

- The invaluable nature of the heart.

- Diet

- Water

- Environmental pollutants

- People at increased risk of particulate matter pollution

- Smokers

- Diabetes and high blood pressure sufferers

- Obesity

- Metabolic syndrome

- Impact of race and ethnicity on cardiovascular disease

- Pause For Thought

- Take Home Nuggets

- Pages for personal notes

A functional heart is an absolute necessity if we are to remain alive. To keep our hearts functional, we need to take every available step to ensure our hearts are kept in optimal health. Unfortunately, our heart health is continually challenged by its exposure to numerous hazards, some of which we are aware of but others we may not.

Diet

In the preceding chapters we alluded to a variety of diets. We mentioned keto diets and Mediterranean-style diets, showing some preference for a Mediterranean-style diet for improved cardiac health. We also spoke of the acquisition of some 10% - 25% of cholesterol from our diets. Our bodies produce some 75% to 90% of all our cholesterol, and we have been told repeatedly that of the two types of cholesterol; HDL is considered as good cholesterol. High levels of HDL above 60mg/dL are associated with heart attacks and death. Universally we are told that LDL is bad cholesterol. Yet we know that cholesterol performs several important roles in our bodies, and LDL in its unoxidized form is not harmful to our hearts. We are continuously treated with drugs which are known to be toxic to try to reduce our cholesterol levels, and in an indirect way protect our hearts, but studies have told us that there is no link between using statins and living longer, and there is no relationship between cholesterol levels and survival rates. We believe, though, that our diets can have a negative impact on our cardiac health, as discussed above.

Water

There are few, if any, communities around the world that have both chlorinated drinking water and a low incidence of cardiovascular disease. High school chemistry students know that chlorine is a powerful oxidising agent. It is because of its oxidising ability that it is a major component of bleach. Extrapolating this information helps us to understand the impact it can have on our blood vessels. In animal studies, chlorine promotes the development of atherosclerosis. In a sort of natural experiment, 75% of American servicemen who were killed fighting in Korea and Vietnam were found to have atherosclerosis. It is alleged that this was because of the chlorine in the water these men drank.

Although our drinking water in the UK also has chlorine, the stated amount is no more than 0.5mg/L. Having said that, it is reasonably easy to free your drinking water from chlorine by simply boiling it for 5 to 10 minutes or by adding a small amount of vitamin C crystals before drinking it.

Environmental pollutants

Research by the Environmental Protection Agency and others have found that exposure to increased concentrations of particulate matter of less than 2.5 micrometres in diameter for hours can trigger cardiovascular disease, such as heart attacks and even death. We are not advising that you should go out and measure the dimension of the particulate matter to which you may be exposed, but we are asking that you be minded that air pollution has been found to contribute to the development of cardiovascular disease. A large body of scientific research has shown that air pollution can exacerbate existing cardiovascular disease and contribute to the development of the disease. The evidence is strongest for outdoor particles. The risk to the individual from particulate matter is smaller than for other well-known risk factors for cardiovascular disease. For the population, though, both short- and long-term exposure has been shown to be associated with increased hospitalisations for serious cardiovascular events, particularly in people with established heart disease.

On exposure to fine particulate matter, people with chronic heart disease may experience palpitations, unusual fatigue, light-headedness, shortness of breath and/or chest tightness or pain in the chest, neck or shoulder, all symptoms of a heart attack.

Possible air contaminants of a diameter less than 2.5 microns include combustion particles, organic compounds, metals etc. Even smaller particles less than 10 microns in diameter including dust, pollen, and mould can impact our cardiac health.

People at increased risk of particulate matter pollution

- People with underlying cardiovascular conditions, for example, ischaemic heart disease and heart failure, or who have previously experienced cardiovascular events such as a stroke or heart attack.
- People with diabetes.
- People with elevated cholesterol levels.
- Non-white populations.
- People who are obese.
- People of low socioeconomic status.
- Older adults.

Of note, wildfire smoke is composed of a mixture of particulate matter including particles less than 2.5 micrometres in diameter. Studies have shown that exposure to wildfire smoke can lead to a variety of health complications in people with underlying lung and heart conditions.

Smokers

I need not tell you that smoking tobacco products, whether you are the primary smoker or one who inhales second-hand smoke, is a leading cause of lung cancer, heart disease and stroke, among other diseases. It is also associated with sudden infant death syndrome and more frequent and severe asthma attacks.

Diabetes and high blood pressure sufferers

People who suffer from either or both conditions are at an increased risk of cardiovascular disease.

The effect of high blood pressure not only results from the heart having to work harder in pumping blood against a greater resistance in the vasculature, but also leads to damage of the walls of the vessels, particularly the arteries which function in carrying blood to tissues away from the heart. The arteries will therefore have to face this higher blood pressure, which can damage the wall of the arteries. The damaged wall of the artery will attract LDL cholesterol to affect a repair. This LDL cholesterol then becomes oxidised, forming a template for atherosclerosis and thus setting up a vicious cycle.

Obesity

One can posit that with obesity the heart must work that much harder because of the increased amount of tissue it must supply. There may be more to this association than simply increased amount of tissue to which the heart must pump blood.

We know that associated with obesity are numerous health challenges: among them is the metabolic syndrome, increased circulating levels of insulin, and this influences our cholesterol levels. There has been much discussion on the effects of cholesterol and heart disease above, so we will not repeat this here. Associated with obesity may be an element of thyroid dysfunction which can also influence the cholesterol milieu and lead to heart disease.

Metabolic syndrome

Metabolic syndrome is the medical term for a combination of diabetes, high blood pressure and obesity. It puts the patient at increased risk of getting coronary heart disease, stroke and other conditions that affect blood vessels.

The insulin resistance which is almost always present in patients with metabolic syndrome will eventually lead to type 2 diabetes and heart and blood vessel disease. The resulting insulin resistance will lead to high levels of cholesterol; add to this high blood pressure and one can easily see the association with the build-up of plaque in the arteries. The plaque narrows and hardens the arteries, leading to a heart attack and/or stroke.

Impact of race and ethnicity on cardiovascular disease

Cardiovascular disease is a leading cause of death in both the United States of America and the United Kingdom. It is found to be more so among ethnic minority groups. The obvious question becomes: Is the white person at a lower risk of heart disease simply because she/he is white or because of other intervening factors?

Researchers tell us that social factors, known as social determinants, of health may be the drivers of the discrepancies that we see among racial lines.

Cardiovascular statistics tell us that 47% of black adults have been diagnosed with cardiovascular disease, compared with 36% of white adults. It also seems that when addressing cardiovascular risk factors, minority groups are more predisposed. For example, Hispanic women are more than twice as likely as white women to have diabetes, a major risk factor for heart disease, as discussed above, while American Indians are three times more likely than whites to have diabetes.

These health differences are not because of genetics, but social factors seem to play a role in shaping people's health. Among these are:

- Money and resources necessary for procuring life's basic needs.
- The quality, standard and exposure to education.
- The quality of the health care they receive.
- The environment in which they live, is clean air and water present?
- Do they have access to fresh fruits and vegetables?

- What is their social existence like? Are they in supportive relationships free of discrimination and violence?

Believe it or not, all these factors can impact our health and have nothing to do with our genetics, but more to do with our social existence.

Pause For Thought

- Can cardiovascular disease be described as multifactorial?
- Does Diet play a role in causing heart disease?
- Can Drinking piped water play a role in the development of cardiovascular disease?
- Are there environmental pollutants that can cause cardiovascular disease?
- Can cardiovascular disease be caused by particulate matter?
- Is race directly related to Cardiovascular disease?

Take Home Nuggets

- Cardiovascular disease is multifactorial, meaning that there are several factors which could affect our cardiovascular system leading to disease. The diet we consume, the water we drink, particularly if it is piped water; dust and other particles in the air can also contribute to damaging our cardiovascular health. Chronic diseases such as diabetes and high blood pressure as well as obesity can influence cardiovascular health. There is an association with one's race but it seems that that relationship is caused by other factors, mainly economic factors.

Notes

Notes

Chapter 7
Blood Pressure

- Normal blood pressure

- Low blood pressure

- High blood pressure

- Types of high blood pressure

- Factors which influence high blood pressure

- The value of treating high blood pressure

- Treatment for high blood pressure

- Other methods of lowering high blood pressure

- Rauvolfia

- Pause For Thought

- Take Home Nuggets

- Pages for personal notes

Every living human being will have a measurable blood pressure which is reported as S/D, where S refers to the systolic value and D the diastolic value. These pressures are generated by the blood flowing through the blood vessels. The systolic blood pressure is defined as the pressure of the blood flow through the arteries during contraction of the heart muscles, while the diastolic blood pressure is defined as the blood pressure generated in the vessels when the heart is resting. To ensure proper blood pressure surveillance, we have identified a blood pressure value considered to be normal. This normal blood pressure is a range of between 90/60 and 120/80. A value considered low, less than 90/60 and one considered high greater than 120/80, and which puts patients at risk of health problems if that pressure is not treated.

Low blood pressure

Low blood pressure, also considered as hypotension, is described as a blood pressure less than 90/60. There are many reasons for this, among which is heavy blood loss and infection. It is important that patients suffering from hypotension should be appropriately treated to ensure that their organs are adequately perfused and thus receive adequate nourishment and oxygen and having the waste products efficiently removed from tissues and organs by the blood flowing through these organs. The usual practice is to increase the fluid available to the patient by providing him or her with intravenous fluids or blood. One needs to be reminded about the rate and volume of fluid infused, and there are guidelines to ensure the safety of this practice. Failure to adequately resuscitate patients with adequate quantities of fluids may have harmful effects on various organs including the kidneys, leading to inadequate production of urine by the kidneys, thereby limiting the ability to excrete waste materials from the body. This would lead to kidney failure and the build-up of waste in our bodies leading to multiple organ failure. If not aggressively treated, this may have disastrous consequences. Blood pressure monitoring therefore becomes inevitable in the presence of procedures that may be associated with heavy blood loss.

High blood pressure

This is a more common finding and is usually diagnosed incidentally or when patients present to their medical personnel with other symptoms. The literature describes high blood pressure as a blood pressure reading of 130/80 or above. In practice, blood pressure readings at 160/90 or above on two or more separate occasions are sufficient to be diagnosed as suffering from high blood pressure. High blood pressure is usually asymptomatic for most parts, though there may be symptoms such as blurred vision, nosebleeds, shortness of breath, chest pains, dizziness, anxiety, palpitations, or the feeling of pulsations in the neck. It may continue to harm you even if there are no symptoms. It is therefore advisable to have your blood pressure checked at regular intervals to ensure that if your blood pressure is high, it can be appropriately treated. If it is high and it remains untreated, then it could lead to irreversible harm to the vessels all over your body, not least in the brain.

Types of high blood pressure

Simply hypertension or high blood pressure can be described as primary or essential hypertension and secondary hypertension. In primary or essential hypertension, there is no obvious known cause or explanation for the high blood pressure; however, there seems to be a familial predisposition (a strong family history of hypertension increases your risk of the condition) and it seems more closely related to age, lifestyle and the environment.

Age seems to be a definite associated factor, as high blood pressure tends to affect individuals more commonly over 50 years of age. It is estimated to affect 63.1% of those over 60 years of age.

Environment may include the quality of our diets and the stresses which we experience daily as we go through life.

Lifestyle may relate to the way in which we lead our lives, the continuous almost habitation of the couch leading to a sedentary lifestyle, as opposed to a more vibrant lifestyle of exploring the open spaces, its relatively fresh, relaxing air and of course the exercise that comes with activity.

In secondary hypertension, there is usually an identifiable cause for the hypertension, maybe some hormonal or glandular dysfunction. There may also be an underlying health condition. There are, however, other triggers that include cigarette smoking, alcohol abuse, obesity, lack of physical activity, diabetes, renal disease, sleep apnoea, thyroid and adrenal gland dysfunction, and birth control tablets.

Factors which influence high blood pressure

There are numerous factors which can influence one's blood pressure. Among them are:

- Viscous (thick blood)
- Sleep apnea
- Renal (kidney) disease
- Low potassium and magnesium intake

- Use of alcohol, caffeine and other stimulants
- Cancer
- Hyperthyroid
- Heavy metal toxicity
- Side effects from certain drugs

The value of treating high blood pressure

Many may ask, seeing that uncontrolled hypertension rarely causes symptoms, is there any need to treat the condition? We in the medical fraternity believe that untreated hypertension is dangerous because it can lead to strokes, heart attacks, heart failure and kidney disease. The goal of treating high blood pressure is to lower this abnormal pressure, and in doing this protect important organs like the brain, heart and kidneys from damage.

With untreated high blood pressure, it increases strain on the heart, causing it to work too hard and thus resulting in a loss of strength. The high force of blood flow which results with untreated high blood pressure can damage the blood vessels, making them weak, inelastic, or narrowed. Over time, uncontrolled high blood can harm several important organs: even the eyes can be adversely affected by uncontrolled high blood pressure.

Blood pressure is determined by the amount of blood the heart pumps and the arteries' resistance to the blood flow. We have noted the effect of high blood pressure on multiple organ systems, even in the absence of symptoms. It is therefore imperative that we must make every effort to maintain our blood pressure within the safe narrow range we consider normal. Excess weight, high-salt diet, stress, and cholesterol are all culprits associated with the development of high blood pressure.

Treatment for high blood pressure

In the scenario above, in which various factors associated with hypertension are mentioned, the appropriate approach would involve dietary changes, exercise, relaxation techniques and/or the use of cholesterol-lowering drugs. Unfortunately, in about 95% of patients suffering from hypertension the cause is unknown, and the steps suggested above may be insufficient to keep the blood pressure within safe limits. Medications may therefore be required; these medications, though, are not without side effects such as dizziness, chronic coughs, muscle cramps, fatigue, and erectile dysfunction.

Other methods of lowering blood pressure

Slow, deep breathing has been useful in lowering blood pressure. So useful has been this natural process that equipment with the objective of lowering blood pressure was developed based on this principle. The RESPERATE works on this principle. It is believed that breathing slowly and deeply from the abdomen helps to reduce blood pressure, because it balances the messages from the nervous system that constricts or relaxes arteries and so helps to control the fight-or-flight stress response. With relaxation and reduction of anxiety, constricted vessels dilate and blood flows more easily.

Although I will list some options which will help to lower your blood pressure, please do not stop taking your blood pressure-lowering medications without first consulting your doctor.

- Calcium at a dose of 500mg twice daily aids transmission along nerves that leads to relaxation of arteries and muscles, hence leading to improved blood flow.

- Coenzyme Q10 at a dose of 300mg per day can be useful. Many people suffering with high blood pressure tends to have low levels of this substance. This substance is also beneficial if you suffer from type 2 diabetes.

- Hawthorn extract at a dose of 250mg three times per day. This substance has a blood-thinning effect and therefore improves blood flow.

- Magnesium at a dose of 250mg twice a day promotes normal neuronal function as well as muscle action facilitating the flow of blood. Fresh vegetable juice by virtue of its potassium content can play a role in lowering blood pressure.

- A traditional cold Spanish vegetable soup called gazpacho is reputed to drop blood pressure by up to 27%.

This beneficial effect is believed to be due to the nutrients it contains from its raw vegetables, namely carotenoids, vitamin C and antioxidants that minimise the damage done by free radicals. The soup is also thought to be effective because of its potassium content.

Rauvolfia

The two most common causes of high blood pressure are being overweight and living under stressful situations. By employing weight loss procedures and effectively losing weight, we can restore normal blood pressure in some adults; additionally, stress reduction can allow one to recover his/ her normal blood pressure.

Other patients do well with chelation therapy, acupuncture or using supplements such as magnesium and fish oil.

Other non-prescription preparations include Rauvolfia serpentina, a commonly used herb obtained from forests in Asia and South America. Rauvolfia serpentina is now gradually replaced by Rauvolfia vomitoria for the same purpose.

Rauvolfia contains several medicinal compounds called alkaloids, of which reserpine is the most studied. Reserpine calms the nervous system and directly lowers blood pressure by relaxing blood vessels. It also appears to block the effect of the stress hormone adrenaline on blood vessels, preventing their constriction. Unfortunately, this substance is no longer used in the USA because of its side effects.

Pause For Thought

- Why is blood pressure measured as S/D?
- What does the S refer too?
- What does the D refer too?
- What is normal blood pressure?

- What is low blood pressure?

- What is high blood pressure?

- What is the significance of blood pressure?

- What are the two main types of high blood pressure?

Take Home Nuggets

- Blood pressure is the force with which the blood is pumped around the body and the force with which it is returned to the heart. When our hearts contract it forces blood from the heart chambers through the blood vessels by a pressure which is represented by the upper number, the S as in the equation above, After the contraction the heart relaxes and enters diastole, a sort of rest or relaxation during which blood is returned to the heart, the measured pressure is labelled as D in the equation above. So, blood pressure is expressed as the systolic pressure/the diastolic pressure.

- The blood pressure value changes over time so it is important to define the blood pressure defined as normal blood pressure.

- •An adult's normal blood pressure ranges between 90/60 and 120/80. It is important that our blood pressure is maintained within the normal range to ensure that our organ systems receive adequate amount of blood and by extension nourishment and that the blood pressure is sufficient to ensure that various products of cell metabolism are carried away from organs system to other areas where they can be excreted from our bodies.

- If our blood pressure falls below 90/60, our tissues may not be adequately perfused and thus nourishment may fail to reach the tissues in adequate supply whilst the waste products of metabolism may not be efficiently removed. This can lead to damage of various organs which if not appropriately addressed could cause the organ to fail to efficiently conduct its function.

- High blood pressure can also lead to damage in various organ systems, not least the brain in which blood vessels may break leading to complications such as strokes. The vessel wall can also be damaged leading to conditions such as aneurysms.

- High blood pressure is commonly described as essential hypertension when a cause has not been identified.

Notes

Notes

_____

_____

_____

_____

_____

_____

_____

_____

_____

_____

_____

_____

_____

_____

_____

_____

_____

_____

_____

_____

_____

Chapter 8
Cardiovascular Disease and Our Created Devils

- The trend seen in cardiovascular disease
- Created devil 1
- Neutralising the effect of artificial light
- Created devil 2
- The bee effect
- Created devil 3
- Created devil 4
- Pause For Thought
- Take Home Nuggets
- Pages for personal notes

Over the past 30 years, deaths and disability from cardiovascular disease have been steadily rising across the world. In 2019, cardiovascular disease, including stroke, was responsible for one-third of all deaths worldwide. It has been reported that there is a heart attack every 34 seconds in America, and there is a death related to heart disease every minute. This data is surely startling and leads us to wonder if man's inventions play a contributing role and how does this happen?

Heart disease is safely described as an epidemic, and during this epidemic the advice given to patients remains agonisingly unchanged: stay on medications, cut the fats and cholesterol, eat lots of fruits and vegetables, exercise, and don't smoke. Unfortunately, this is the same advice which has been given over several years, and the incidence of the disease is still rising.

Created Devil 1

As children growing up, although we may not have been told, we assumed that night time was for sleeping. It was and may be still difficult to understand why we feel sleepy at nights. The answer may be all related to the secretion of a substance called melatonin by our brains. This substance secretion increases in natural darkness.

Creations emitting artificial light, specifically blue light, as an integral part of their function may contribute to a lower level of melatonin secreted by our brains and thereby, interfere with our sleep. We continue to light up our environments with artificial lighting. We have moved away from being outdoor creatures to being indoor creatures. Our biology has not changed to accommodate this new change. Artificial light, specifically the blue spectrum of this light, immediately destroys melatonin.

Melatonin is a hormone produced by the pineal gland of the brain. This hormone secretion begins at the setting of the sun, and its secretion increases about three hours before our bedtime. The significance of this is that melatonin makes us sleepy: it is responsible for a good night's sleep. Without natural darkness melatonin levels do not rise and this can cause one to have trouble falling asleep and enjoying a restful night's sleep.

Melatonin function is not only to facilitate sleep, but also important for the functioning of the immune system, and it is also a powerful antioxidant. This conclusion is borne out by many research studies which indicate that people who do night work and are continually exposed to artificial light have a far greater incidence of heart disease and stroke. Studies also show that a person working at night reduces their lifespan by about 6 years. Artificial light is also associated with an elevated risk of cancer, diabetes, obesity, depression and sleep disorders.

Neutralising the effect of artificial light

Sun exposure between 6 am and noon has the effect of setting the circadian timing in the suprachiasmatic nucleus of the brain better than any other method.

The superchiasmatic nucleus is a collection of neurons located in the hypothalamus and is the master clock that controls our circadian rhythm. The sun exposure suggested above, should be undertaken with adequate skin and eye exposure without sunscreen or sunglasses.

One practice that may prevent artificial light from interfering with your health is to avoid exposure to artificial light for approximately 3 hours before retiring to bed at night. Additionally, candles, kerosene lamps, fires or the moon do not have significant blue light and are therefore safer. As an adjunct, you may choose to use blue light-blocking glasses at night.

You can liaise with your doctor to determine whether your reduced exposure to blue light has made any impact on your health by having a blood test assessing your high-sensitivity CRP, a measure of inflammation, and sulfated DHEA which is a hormone marker for an inflammatory cytokine, interleukin 6.

Created Devil 2
Electromagnetic fields

We seem to live in an envelope of man-created electromagnetic fields, that almost appear inescapable. With development we have created health challenges. Most would select the lifestyle that we have grown comfortable with but are we sacrificing our health for these conveniences? The Wi-Fi, cell phones, cell towers, broadcast towers, powerlines, wireless features, cars, computers, smart meters, wireless routers, baby monitors and other electronic devices all demonstrate my observation that we have chosen to live in a sea of created electromagnetic radiation with a deleterious effect on our general and cardiac health and disturbing our environment.

The earth has its own electromagnetic field: does the created man-made electromagnetic field have any effect on the earth's electromagnetic field? I hear you ask. The response can quickly be had by just thinking that the effect of the man-made electromagnetic field can either be an accentuation or an antagonising contrary effect.

The bee effect

In a simple experiment in which a cordless phone was placed in a beehive to study the effect and resultant behaviour of the bees, it was found that the bees deserted their hive, and none returned to the hive the following day. Is it any wonder that there has been a drastic decline in honeybees with colony collapse disorder?

As much as 3% of the population are sensitive to electromagnetic fields and become symptomatic when exposed. Studies have shown increased abnormal heartbeat patterns with exposure to electromagnetic fields.

Electromagnetic field exposure has been linked in both animal and human studies to hyperactivity, and learning and behaviour problems. Effects on other aspects of our health are seen in a negative effect on our memory, our learning, our behaviour, attention, sleep disruption, cancer, and neurological diseases like Alzheimer's.

Created Devil 3

The common practice of using statins to reduce cholesterol. We are led to believe that statins, is the answer to lowering our cholesterol. There are seven different statins licensed for use in the USA and five different statins licensed for use in the UK. They are promoted as drugs which are supposed to lower cholesterol by lowering the bad cholesterol (LDL) whilst increasing the good cholesterol (HDL). This explanation has been widely accepted and so the drug seems almost a knee-jerk necessity for anyone who has had a heart attack and/or stroke. It has been reported that more than 70 million prescriptions are dispensed for statins in England each year.

It must be understood that our bodies, through the liver, produce 75–90% of all the cholesterol our body needs. The amount of cholesterol obtained from our diets contributes a mere 10%–25%. It would therefore seem, realistically, that the amount of cholesterol obtained through our diets makes only a small difference to our total cholesterol load. We are told that the way in which statins produce their effect is through the blockage of the enzyme in the liver which produces cholesterol.

But we know now that statins will not lengthen your lifespan and may kill you, rendering them as an effective slow poison. The literature is replete with cases of side effects of statins, muscle cramps, sleep disturbances and the inability to walk, as well as other features associated with muscle weakness, leading to disability. Research has indicated that statins can lead to early death.

In an experiment conducted by Duke University, researchers caring for the elderly who were on statins and who they thought had less than a year to live, to save money discontinued the use of statins in half of these patients. They were surprised to note that those in the group who were taken off statins lived on average 40 days longer than those kept on statins. A study in Expert Reviews in Clinical Pharmacology in 2015, captioned "Statins stimulate atherosclerosis (narrowing of arteries) and heart failure: Pharmacological mechanisms", reported that statins lower coenzyme Q10 and decrease cell energy production, which is bad news for the heart and brain, both of which need a lot of energy. Statins also inhibit the synthesis of vitamin K2 which prevents calcification of arteries and other soft tissues. Finally, the researchers believe that they have found the underlying cause of the cardiovascular disease epidemic which statins tend to encourage by inhibiting the biosynthesis of selenium containing proteins. Statins therefore are not saving your heart, but they may be damaging it permanently.

Created Devil 4

The explanation for adding chlorine to drinking water is to disinfect the water. Chlorine is able to kill bacteria, viruses, and other disease-causing organisms (pathogens). The typical rationale given is that the addition of chlorine is effective and continues to keep the water safe as it travels from the treatment plant to the consumer.

Whilst that may be so, we see several relatively new diseases arise, and it leads one to wonder whether we are contributing to the development of the various diseases from which we suffer.

Going back to my days as a chemistry student, it does not fail to register that chlorine is among the strongest known oxidising agents. It occupies a position high in the electrochemical series, a chart which places substances in order of their ability to oxidise matter. Let us keep it simple, since chlorine is among the most powerful oxidising agents known, and we have learned above that LDL cholesterol is deadliest in oxidised form: can we now see the link between chlorine in our drinking water and heart disease? Chlorine thus can oxidise LDL cholesterol which thus produces its effect on the blood vessels, generating plaque and promoting atherosclerosis, with its deadly sequelae.

Pause For Thought

- Are we guilty of producing environmental effects which are harmful to our hearts?
- Does blue light have any effect on cardiovascular health?
- Does electromagnetic radiation have any effect on cardiovascular health?
- Does electromagnetic radiation have any effect on bees?
- Do statins have an adverse effect on our cardiovascular health?

Take Home Nuggets

- With the advent of the blue light, from our mobile phones, our TV's our computers, we find it more difficult to drift off to sleep, since our melatonin levels have not increased sufficiently to allow us to have the deep relaxing sleep which we had prior to the advent of this sea of blue light in our homes. Additionally, we seem to be living in an electromagnetic bubble with the wifi's, mobile devices etc, this too has impacted our cardiovascular health. Bees were noted to vacate their hives and not return when a mobile phone was placed in their hives. Unfortunately, statins which are widely prescribed as medications designed to improve our cardiac health, have also been shown to increase the risk of cardiovascular disease.

Notes

Notes

Chapter 9
Healing Your Heart

- Steps to reversing your heart disease
  - ○ Step 1: Sunlight
  - ○ Step 2: Magnesium
  - ○ Step 3: Coenzyme
  - ○ Step 4: Omega-3 fatty acid DHA
  - ○ Step 5: Vitamin K2
- The shocking findings
  - ○ Other useful test which are more sensitive in predicting cardiac disease
  - ○ Second useful test
  - ○ Third useful test
  - ○ The fourth useful test
- Pause For Thought
- Take Home Nuggets
- Pages for personal notes

Steps to reversing your heart disease

We go as our cardiovascular system allows us. If we have poor heart health, we will invariably be poorly. It is therefore vital that our heart health is optimised as safely as possible. Yet we see in the previous chapter that we tend to be repeating our practice without any improvement in outcome. Case in point: half of the world's bypass and stent procedures are performed on Americans, and about 30% of adults over the age of 40 are on cholesterol-lowering statins, yet the incidence of cardiovascular disease and death because of cardiovascular disease continues to rise, at least in the USA, which still has the highest rate of heart disease in the world, and cardiovascular deaths are on the rise.

This is hardly surprising because research tells us that statins do not extend lives, neither does angioplasties, stents, and coronary bypass surgeries. Yet we do not seem to be learning because we keep recommending the same practice and the same procedures.

Is it time to explore a different approach?

Let us take a 5 step-journey to try to reverse a diseased heart.

Step 1: Sunlight

Step 1 appears to be based on common sense: we advocate that you should get plenty of sunlight. Ensuring a plentiful supply of sun on your skin daily is by far the cheapest way to reduce your risk of cardiovascular disease. Researchers tell us that women who got regular sun exposure lived 1–2 years longer than those who did not. The explanation for this difference was based on the reduction in cardiovascular events such as heart attack and stroke in the exposed group.

- It has been found that sunlight causes the production of sulfated cholesterol in the skin. This compound helps in protecting against heart attack.

Sulfated cholesterol also keeps our red blood cell membranes supple and pliable so that they can squeeze through the tiny capillaries in our circulatory system.

- Sulfated cholesterol also repairs damage of the inner lining of our arteries, consequently reducing plaque formation and build-up.

- It is also water-soluble and so can travel to all tissues of the body. Additionally, it is converted to sulfated vitamin D which is beneficial in reducing cardiovascular disease.

Step 2: Magnesium

The use of magnesium and its positive role in heart health cannot be overstated. Magnesium is critical to most enzymes which are involved in energy production. I need not tell you that the heart muscle has a high need for energy.

Magnesium also has additional benefits in that it has been shown to inhibit blood clots, block calcium uptake, thin the blood and relax blood vessels. Low magnesium is associated with elevated blood pressure, a known risk factor for heart attacks and strokes.

Unfortunately, the magnesium content in our foods has been declining; coupled with that, 80–95% of total magnesium is removed in the processing of grains. Depending on our regular foods to give us adequate amounts of magnesium may be failing us, and for this reason there is a need to consider supplementation with magnesium. Of the various magnesium supplements available, those with the greatest absorbance are: magnesium malate, which increases endurance; magnesium taurate, which helps the heart; magnesium glycinate, which increases the availability of energy; magnesium citrate, which is best absorbed in the body and improves digestion; and magnesium threonate, which is only a recent preparation but has been shown to penetrate the energy factories of the cells, that is the mitochondria, and has been shown to cross the blood-brain barrier.

Step 3: Coenzyme Q10

Studies have shown that coenzyme Q10 supplementation improves heart function, reduces the risk of cardiovascular disease, reverses the symptoms of heart failure, and is protective of the brain by preventing brain degeneration. Like magnesium it also plays a role in energy production.

Unfortunately, this useful substance level declines with aging, hence the need for supplementation. The preferred formulation for this substance taken as a supplement is ubiquinol, as it is better absorbed through the gastrointestinal tract and works more efficiently in the mitochondria to improve cellular energy.

Step 4: Omega-3 fatty acid DHA

Omega−3 fatty acid, DHA, is abundant in seafood and plays a critical role in the reduction of cardiovascular disease. Low levels of DHA greatly increase the risk of cardiovascular disease. Processed foods are a major culprit in depleting 'our bodies supply of DHA. DHA supplementation can be had, or it can be obtained from the diet which includes wild caught salmon, sardines, trout cod and shellfish, which has the added benefit of containing sulphur. This sulphur can be used for sulfation of cholesterol and vitamin D.

Step 5: Vitamin K2

Heart health is dependent on vitamin K2. The Rotterdam Study involving nearly 5,000 people informed us that participants who ingested the greatest quantities of vitamin K2 in their diet experience a 57% reduction in death from heart disease compared to the cohort of patients who ingested the least vitamin K2.

Vitamin K2 plays the critical role in preventing calcium from building up in the walls of arteries. Calcium in the arteries is deadly, as it leads to the build-up of plaque and thus restricts blood flow.

There are two types of vitamin K2: MK-4 and MK-7.

MK-4 is found in certain animal foods, such as dark red meat of chicken, goose liver pâté and raw, grass-fed dairy. The difficulty with MK-4 is it only stays in the body for a few hours.

MK-7, on the other hand, stays in your body for days. It is found in fermented foods such as natto and cheese like French Brie, Jarlsberg from Norway, Swiss Emmental and Dutch Edam. It is advisable that a supplement containing both MK-4 and MK-7 be used.

Doctors continue to treat patients for cardiovascular diseases by placing them on prophylactic medications, yet patients continue to suffer from cardiovascular illnesses, so do our management and prophylactic efforts need a review?

The shocking findings

There are two shocking findings which suggest that our management needs a review:

(1)   About 50% of people who have their first heart attack have normal cholesterol. This therefore suggests that screening for cholesterol levels is a poor predictor of subsequent cardiovascular events.

(2)   Most heart attacks occur when a piece of plaque lining an artery breaks off and causes a blockage downstream: this leads to a sudden heart attack if the blockage occurs in the coronary vessels. This points to a deficiency with standard cardiac testing.

The usual care afforded to patients fails to account for these two important facts:

1. The usual cardiac stress test is failed when the tested patient has a pre-existing blockage of one of the arteries supplying blood to the heart, but if you do not have occlusive disease of your heart arteries you may pass the stress test and, occasionally, are erroneously told you have a clean bill of health.

2. The other commonly offered test is called a lipid profile but as indicated above, about 50% of cardiac attack victims have normal lipid profiles.

Other useful blood tests which are more sensitive in predicting cardiac disease

Testing for lipoprotein A; lipoprotein A is a dangerous little molecule with a corkscrew tail which makes it particularly dangerous. It is a compound that is present in all of us, but when it is at a high concentration it is particularly dangerous. Of note, the levels of this substance can be high when the regular lipid profile numbers fall within normal range. Epidemiological studies have identified lipoprotein (a) as a risk factor for artherosclerosis and related cardiovascular diseases.

Second useful test

We have spoken at length about good cholesterol, high-density lipoprotein cholesterol (HDL) and bad cholesterol low-density lipoprotein cholesterol (LDL). But LDL is not as dangerous as the oxidised form which induces both atherosclerosis and plaque formation and hardens the arterial walls. Increased levels of oxidised LDL which can be determined by a blood test point to the presence of coronary heart disease. The levels of this substance are particularly useful, since the higher the level, the worse the cardiac disease; it can also be used as a measure to determine if your treatment is working.

Third useful test

Checking the levels of lipoprotein-associated phospholipase 2 is an essential test which is not readily done by doctors. It is a measure of the stability of plaque.

This is an important test because inflamed unstable cardiac plaque is more likely to rupture, break off and cause a sudden heart attack.

The fourth useful test

This test differs from the previous three which were blood tests, this test is an imaging study called the carotid intima-media thickness (CIMT). Data reveals that a CIMT increment of 0.1mm increases the risk of a heart attack by 10–15% and the risk of a stroke by 13–18%. This very useful test is safe, non-invasive and can be done over five minutes. It can therefore be used repeatedly to determine whether treatment is working or not. The CIMT also gives an indication of early disease. It is a simple ultrasound study which measures artery wall thickness and plaque build-up. By performing the CIMT ultrasound one can determine whether methods employed for the reversal of cardiac disease is actually working.

Through these tests we can monitor cardiac disease development and progress, and by employing the five steps listed in this chapter we may be better able to arrest the epidemic of cardiovascular disease.

Pause For Thought

- Are there any options available to us to improve and reclaim our cardiovascular health?
- Can sunlight play a role in us regaining our cardiovascular health?
- Are there any supplements available to help me regain my cardiovascular health?

- Is there a specific blood test which can measure my risk of cardiovascular disease?

- Can I measure the stability of plaque in my blood vessels?

- Is there a non-invasive test available for determining the risk for cardiovascular disease?

Take Home Nuggets

- Although we are guilty of creating an environment which can adversely affect our cardiovascular health, we note the importance of sunlight in facilitating cardiovascular health. Supplements of the type coenzyme Q 10 and omega 3 fatty acid DHA, vitamin K2 are all useful supplements.

- There are also some tests which allows us to determine how successful we are in improving cardiovascular health. Testing for lipoprotein associated phospholipase 2 gives an indication of the stability of plaque.

Notes

Notes

_____

_____

_____

_____

_____

_____

_____

_____

_____

_____

_____

_____

_____

_____

_____

_____

_____

_____

_____

_____

_____

Chapter 10
The Little-Mentioned Heart Attack Risks: Poor Circulation, Thick Blood, Failure to Brush your Teeth and Homocysteine are Related

- Poor circulation

- Symptoms of poor circulation

- Help for poor circulation.

- Thick blood

- Causes

- Symptoms of thick blood

- Significance of thick blood

- Some possible effects of blood clots

- Medical options for treatment

- Non-medical options

- Brush your teeth

- The homocysteine threat.

- Pause For Thought

- Take Home Nuggets

- Pages for personal notes

What do poor circulation, thick blood, failure to brush one's teeth and homocysteine have in common? These apparently unrelated entities are all linked by the ability to induce cardiovascular disease.

Poor circulation

When blood circulation is impaired, it causes the build-up of fluid over time. This accumulation of fluid is called oedema and can be an early sign of heart failure due to the heart not being able to adequately provide oxygen and other nourishment all around the body. This can lead to the formation of blood clots which can be deadly. Peripheral artery disease can increase your risk of a heart attack. Poor blood circulation may be a manifestation of broader health issues. It must be realised that your entire body depends on a healthy circulatory system to keep organs properly supplied with oxygen.

Symptoms of poor circulation

Symptoms of poor circulation include swelling of extremities, particularly the dependent extremities, muscle cramping, constant foot pain, pains and throbbing in the arms and legs, fatigue, varicose veins, and digestive issues.

Leg cramps while walking and wounds that don't heal in your legs and toes are also symptoms. Confusion and forgetfulness may also be a manifestation of diminished blood supply and oxygen to the brain. Poor circulation can lead to death of the involved body part. The skin may appear pale or blue because of lack of blood flow.

Help for poor circulation

(1) Compression devices, such as thromboembolic deterrent stockings for dependent extremities where the excess fluid is likely to accumulate. This is non-invasive and should be the first-choice option.

(2) There are units which offer compression therapy who advise that this type of therapy not only increases circulation, but can also allow you to maintain your full range of motion.

(3) Ginkgo biloba.

Ginkgo extract can help at a dose of 120mg twice daily for about eight weeks. It is believed to bring about dilation of the arteries in the limbs and so improve circulation. With the arteries dilated it means that more blood can be brought to the limbs which would in effect carry nutrients and oxygen to the limbs and simultaneously remove waste from the involved tissues. Additionally, there is less resistance to blood flow which could be positively beneficial to your blood pressure and the work expected of the heart.

(4) Nattokinase.

An enzyme detected through mere coincidence in 1980 by a Japanese researcher called Hiroyuki Sumi at the Chicago University Medical School while he was in search of a substance capable of dissolving blood clots. This enzyme is the by-product of fermented boiled soya beans. It is considered a natural blood thinner. You should not take this preparation unless you first discuss it with your doctor, particularly if you are on other blood- thinning agents. Nattokinase dissolves blood clots, hence maintaining good blood vessel wall integrity and improving blood flow, reducing the risk of heart disease. By extension, it can lower blood pressure and improve artery health. There is also evidence that nattokinase lowers the risk of blood clot formation during long-haul travel.

Because of its known mechanism of action, caution is advised when using this preparation in conjunction with other blood thinners. One should also avoid this preparation if going into theatre for any type of surgery, for two reasons: (a) the anaesthetist will have difficulty controlling your blood pressure; and (b) its blood-thinning properties may make haemostasis challenging for the surgeon. As we have always made clear, before embarking on any preparation, we suggest talking to your doctor first.

Thick blood

The term 'thick blood' is also referred to in medical parlance as polycythaemia. This term literally means having an excess of red blood cells in your blood. With thick blood, the blood is less able to flow through blood vessels and organs. This sluggish flow is not without symptoms and complications.

Causes

Among the various causes of thick blood are:

(1) Excess blood cells in circulation (as in chronic leukaemia)

(2) Diseases which affect blood clotting (as in factor V Leiden deficiency)

(3) Excess clotting proteins in the blood, of which there are two types:

(a) acquired (the more common type, seen in smokers, obese individuals and pregnancy); and (b) the genetic or inherited type such as in patients with protein S deficiency.

Symptoms of thick blood

- Blurred vision
- Dizziness
- Easy bruising
- In women, excessive menstrual bleeding
- Gout
- Headache
- High blood pressure
- Itchy skin

Significance of thick blood

The significance of having thick blood is that it puts the individual at increased risk of excessive clotting, or clotting when you are not bleeding.

Some possible effects of blood clots

- A stroke. There are two types of stroke. In the thrombotic or ischaemic stroke, a blood clot prevents blood flow distal to it, so the organs and tissues downfield from the clot is starved of oxygen and nutrients, whilst the waste produced is not removed. In a haemorrhagic stroke, a blood vessel ruptures so there is bleeding from the vessel with similar consequences as in the thrombotic stroke. When this clot occurs in blood vessels supplying the brain, a stroke results.

- If the clot occurs in the vessels supplying the heart, a heart attack results.
- A blood clot in the kidney arteries can lead to kidney failure.
- A blood clot in the lungs, called a pulmonary embolus, can lead to chest pains, difficulty breathing and even death.
- A blood clot in the veins in your arm or leg can cause pain, swelling, redness or increased warmth in the affected limb and even death of the affected limb. The clot can also break off and travel to the lungs where it can cause a pulmonary embolus.
- Clots in the blood vessels can give rise to the narrowing of arteries leading to peripheral artery disease. This may lead to pain in the legs whilst walking or running.
- Believe it or not, blood clots can have deleterious effects in pregnancy, not only for the mother, but also for the wellbeing of the foetus: for example, blood clots may lead to miscarriages, still births and pregnancy-related complications such as pre-eclampsia.

It is therefore imperative that we treat thick blood to minimise some of these unpleasant effects.

Medical options for treatment

The treatment for thick blood may take one of three approaches:

(a) Antiplatelet therapy may be used, so drugs like aspirin by reducing the stickiness of platelets can help prevent platelets from clumping together to form clots.

(b) Anticoagulation therapy can be used. Some drugs, such as warfarin, act on coagulation factors and thereby prevent blood clots from being formed.

(c) Thrombolytics: these clot-busting preparations, such as streptokinase, are used in emergency situations under medical care.

There should be no doubt as to the usefulness of treating thick blood. In fact, Dr Gregory Sloop from Louisiana State University School of Medicine at New Orleans suggests that all the major factors for atherosclerosis ultimately damage blood vessels because of the associated blood thickness.

In the Edinburgh Artery Study involving 4,860 men between the ages of 45 and 59, and women aged between 55 and 74 years, it was found that the 20% of the study participants with the thickest and stickiest blood had 55% of the major cardiovascular events over a five-year period. It has been shown that the link between thick blood and cardiovascular events was as strong as diastolic blood pressure and LDL cholesterol, and stronger than the risk caused by smoking. It therefore advances the case for treatment of thick, sticky blood as aggressively as possible. Furthermore, in a study reported in the European Journal of Clinical

Investigation, the researchers found that men in a group with the thickest blood had more than a three- fold risk of cardiovascular events such as a heart attack or stroke.

It is important to note that the thickness and stickiness of blood vary with the phase of the heartbeat. During cardiac contraction, the phenomenon called systole. The blood is less thick and sticky. During diastole, when the heart relaxes as represented by the D in the blood pressure reading, the thickness and stickiness of blood can be increased by a factor of 20.

Non-medical options

It therefore seems that the combination of high blood pressure and blood thickness is a dangerous one. So whatever method can be safely used to treat the blood pressure, as well as reduce blood stickiness, should be encouraged.

We have been encouraged to donate blood repeatedly to save the life of others who may need it, but there is hardly any mention of benefit to the donor. Among the benefits to the donor is the reduction in the stickiness of the rest of your blood, as well as a reduction in your blood pressure. Other benefits include creation of younger and more flexible red blood cells.

Drinking adequate volumes of water to keep you hydrated also helps in the reduction of the thickness of blood. Most people need between 50 (1.5 litres) and 80 (2.4 litres) ounces of water daily, depending on their physical activity.

Fish oil supplements (as well as eating fish) are also useful because of their high content of EPA and DHA which among other things, reduce your cardiovascular risk by decreasing blood thickness and stickiness.

Another useful option is the use of nattokinase which not only dissolves blood clots on contact, but also has been shown to reduce blood pressure and reduce the risk of osteoporosis.

Brush your teeth

The data is frightening. Researchers from University College London found that individuals who brushed their teeth less than twice per day had a 70% increased risk of heart disease compared to those who brushed at least twice per day.

The homocysteine threat

Homocysteine is an amino acid that promotes the growing of smooth muscle cells just below the lining of the blood vessels. If the homocysteine levels become too high, they encourage the rapid growth of these underlying smooth muscle cells which create a bulge in the vessel. It is on this bulge that the bad cholesterol, blood products like platelets and calcium, accumulates. This accumulation leads to problems like impotence, poor memory, heart attacks and even strokes.

A Seattle team of researchers working with baboons were able to show that injections with homocysteine resulting in high levels caused early signs of atherosclerosis in their experimental animals. After one week of high homocysteine levels about 23% of the animals' arterial wall was lost. The higher the levels of homocysteine, the more severely injured will the arterial wall become and the more severe atherosclerosis.

Interestingly, your body produces homocysteine from an amino acid called methionine which is present in all animal and plant proteins. Through digestion the methionine is converted to homocysteine. Under normal circumstances and in the presence of certain additional substances such as vitamin B6, vitamin B12 and folic acid, the homocysteine is converted into harmless products.

It is difficult to acquire healthy levels of B6, B12 and folate from your diet only, so, as such, supplementation becomes essential. Many health food stores may have a homocysteine formula containing vitamin B6, vitamin B12 and folate. This preparation may prove useful in lowering your homocysteine levels. This could be a lifesaver.

Pause For Thought

- We have discussed the factors of the heart and vessels which contribute to cardiovascular disease, but are there any features of the blood which can lead to cardiovascular disease?
- Can poor circulation cause or contribute to cardiovascular disease?
- Is there any help for poor circulation?
- Are there any symptoms of poor circulation?
- Is there something called thick blood?
- Are there any symptoms of thick blood?

Take Home Nuggets

- The cardiovascular system is composed of the pump (the heart), the channels (the blood vessels), and the fluid which is pumped by the pump through the channels. Any of the components of the cardiovascular system can lead to dysfunction which causes cardiovascular disease.

- Sluggish blood flow may result if the blood is too thick or maybe because the individual is dehydrated. There are some definite symptoms associated with poor circulation and the blood being too thick. There are both mechanical and nonmechanical options to reduce the effect on the cardiovascular health.

Notes

_____

_____

_____

_____

_____

_____

_____

_____

_____

_____

_____

_____

_____

_____

_____

_____

_____

_____

Notes

Chapter 11
The Metabolic Syndrome

- Syndrome X

- Causes

- Symptoms

- Risks of metabolic syndrome

- Treating metabolic syndrome

- Bergamot story

- Lifestyle changes

- Environmental factors

- Pause For Thought

- Take Home Nuggets

- Pages for personal notes

This is also referred to as syndrome X or insulin resistance syndrome. Essentially this is a collection of conditions that can increase the risk of developing heart disease, stroke, and diabetes. It includes several risk factors, including high blood pressure, high blood sugar, excess body fat around the midline and abnormal cholesterol levels. From the constellation of associated factors, individuals with this condition are at an extremely high risk of developing cardiovascular disease.

Although this is not a disease but a condition which is a collection of risk factors, if untreated it can lead to an individual developing serious health problems.

This constellation of symptoms is more prevalent than one could imagine, as one in four adults in the USA has at least three of these risk factors.

Causes

Three major causes of the metabolic syndrome are genetics, lifestyle, and environmental factors.

Genetically it seems that some individuals are more prone to developing the condition than others.

Lifestyle factors such as poor, unhealthy diets, and a sedentary lifestyle contribute to the development of this syndrome.

Environmental factors such as environmental toxins can contribute to the development of this condition.

Symptoms

Though the symptoms resulting from this condition are person-dependent, the more commonly seen symptoms include:

- Elevated blood pressure
- Elevated blood sugar levels
- Abnormal cholesterol levels

- Insulin resistance
- Truncal obesity

Having one or two of these symptoms may not be enough to place you in the category of suffering from metabolic syndrome, but it is always advisable to discuss with your attending doctor if you think that you may be having this problem.

Risks of metabolic syndrome

As stated above, metabolic syndrome places an individual in a high- risk category for the development of certain health conditions. With this syndrome, an individual is at increased risk of developing heart disease, stroke, Alzheimer's disease, dementia, and diabetes.

They are also at increased risk of developing breast and colon cancers.

Treating metabolic syndrome

With a constellation of symptoms which can lead to these life-threatening conditions like heart disease, stroke, Alzheimer's, dementia, cancer and diabetes, aggressive treatment of this condition will help to reduce the incidence of these life-threatening conditions.

Some suggest a keto diet which would effectively force the body to use up its fats as its energy-producing fuel, hence reducing the fat stored, the triglyceride levels and the LDL (bad cholesterol). Nature has, however, provided us with an interesting alternative in the citrus fruit bergamot.

Bergamot story

Bergamot is a citrus fruit with the colour of lemon, but the size of a medium to large orange. As a citrus fruit, it is less sour than lemon but much more bitter than grapefruit.

Why torture your taste buds with this fruit? I hear you ask, and the simple answer is because of the tremendous benefits it presents. In just 30 days, it drops LDL cholesterol by 37%, triglycerides by 49%, and blood sugar levels by up to 22%. These results are particularly significant when compared to the results produced by statins with the associated adverse effects; with bergamot you will only have to cope with its bitter taste.

Bergamot is believed to bring about its effect in a similar manner to statins by blocking one of the enzymes, HMG-CoA reductase, which is necessary for cholesterol production. Bergamot is particularly useful in treating the metabolic syndrome because with the metabolic syndrome there is an association with insulin resistance and consequently high sugar levels. The enzyme HMG-CoA activity increases when blood sugar levels are high.

Bergamot components also have an impact on high blood sugar levels by acting directly on glucose transporter proteins and glucose-regulating enzymes, as well as increasing insulin sensitivity, thus reducing blood sugar levels. Bergamot components also have powerful antioxidant properties which help to maintain good health.

The key components of bergamot are a group of flavonoids which include:

- Naringin

- Rutin

- Narirutin

- Hesperidin

- Neoeriocitrin

- Eriocitrin

- Neohesperidin

Of these components, naringin has been the most extensively studied. As it turns out, naringin, a super-powerful bioflavonoid, is the source of this fruit's bitterness. This bioflavonoid has been shown in multiple studies to lower high cholesterol, triglycerides and blood sugar levels.

One study has shown that naringin by itself was able to lower LDL cholesterol by 17% and total cholesterol by 14% in patients struggling with high cholesterol.

Studies of high blood sugar levels, a symptom of the metabolic syndrome, showed that when naringin is combined with hesperidin, they bring about a lowering of blood sugar levels, a vital step in protecting individuals from developing type 2 diabetes.

Additionally, naringin can reduce triglycerides levels and thus optimise cardiovascular health.

Whereas the symptoms of metabolic syndrome, including elevated blood pressure, low HDL cholesterol (good cholesterol), elevated triglyceride levels, elevated C-reactive protein level, insulin resistance and excessive abdominal fat present an almost inescapable formula for premature death, with bergamot there is hope of being able to reduce this risk.

In the bergamot polyphenolic extract study in which the extracts of bergamot were compared to placebo, 238 patients with high cholesterol and some with high blood sugar were followed for 30 days. In this short period, the patients in the bergamot extract group had cholesterol levels up to 38% lower than those in the placebo group. The results were most impressive in the subgroup of patients who were classed as having the metabolic syndrome. In this group, the patients had a drop of about 49% in their triglyceride levels, and an average drop of 22% in their blood sugar levels.

As indicated above, the bergamot fruit is not enticing to the taste buds, and this is therefore a deterrent to its use. This has been addressed with the formation of a preparation called citrus bergamot. It is recommended that one should take 2–4 tablets daily, before dinner on an empty stomach for 30 days, then a maintenance dose of one capsule daily again before dinner on an empty stomach, to get similar benefits as trying to consume the bitter-tasting fruit.

Lifestyle changes

We have been informed of how dangerous the metabolic syndrome is and that within its complications is a recipe for early or premature death. As a result, it is imperative that we do all we can to avoid this deadly syndrome. We talk of lifestyle changes: this not only considers the volumes we consume, but also cautiously advises us on being more selective in our food choices. A keto diet plan has been recommended with the rationale that it encourages our bodies to use up fats as the primary energy source as opposed to carbohydrates. The accompanying weight loss will not only help in reducing our truncal fat, but also improve our body's sensitivity to insulin, thus helping to keep type 2 diabetes at bay.

Coupled with our selective diet plan, we encourage activity and moving away from a sedentary lifestyle. Our increased physical activity will complement the weight loss induced by our chosen diet, and it will also facilitate our circulation, reducing the probability of developing thick blood and thereby reducing the probability of developing a blood clot.

Environmental factors

The environmental factors leading to metabolic syndrome may arise from exposure to heavy metals, and for this we recommend chelation therapy which can now be achieved with oral preparations, although the parenteral approach is still practised and may be more effective.

Pause For Thought

- What is the metabolic syndrome?
- Are there any causes of the metabolic syndrome?
- Are there any symptoms of the metabolic syndrome?
- How does this affect a patient?
- Are there any treatments?

- Can Bergamot and life style changes help to protect against this condition?

Take Home Nuggets

Metabolic syndrome is an insulin resistance syndrome which is associated with several diseases. Type 2 diabetes, high blood pressure, and obesity are among the more common diseases found in patients with the metabolic syndrome. By extension it is also a risk factor for cardiovascular disease. The impact of this condition can be lessened with lifestyle changes and with the use of bergamot.

Notes

Notes

Chapter 12
Defeating the Heart Attack Enzyme

- Is there a heart attack enzyme?

- Addressing excessive LDL in circulation

- The heart attack enzyme

- Heart attack enzyme busters

- The silk fruit

- Hibiscus

- Garlic

- Foods rich in fibre

- Other useful foods

- Red yeast rice

- Bergamot

- Niacin

- Niacin warning

- Pause For Thought

- Take Home Nuggets

- Pages for personal notes

Much of this book has been discussing the effect of high cholesterol on our cardiovascular system. In summary, we have learned about good cholesterol, or

HDL, which functions, in a nutshell, in reducing the levels of the bad cholesterol, or LDL, in circulation. Yet we learn that up to 90% of the cholesterol in our bodies is made in our liver and intestines. The baffling question becomes: why does our body produce this substance, if it is harmful to us? We have also learned that LDL is not harmful; on the contrary, it is useful, but it is a specialised form of LDL which is harmful and that is the oxidised form of LDL. Simply put, for the LDL to be oxidised it needs to be present; it therefore comes down to the levels of LDL in our system and how can its oxidation be prevented.

We know that LDL has several uses in our bodies, and this therefore explains why our body synthesises 75–90% of its cholesterol needs; that is, our body produces both HDL (good cholesterol) and LDL (bad cholesterol). LDL is more abundantly produced than HDL. Whereas HDL clears LDL from our bodies, LDL is utilised in our bodies to produce hormones such as testosterone, oestrogen, and cortisol. LDL is necessary to produce vitamin D; it is involved in metabolic processes and forms an integral part of the cell membrane. LDL is necessary and plays a vital role in the normal functioning of our bodies. LDL is produced in our livers and intestines through the activity of an enzyme called HMG-CoA reductase. Unfortunately, as we age, this enzyme level and activity fluctuates, leading to higher-than-normal levels of LDL; additionally, as we age, our bodies have reduced needs for LDL to produce hormones. We know that in the menopause the amount of oestrogen in circulation declines; similarly, as men get older the amount of circulating testosterone declines, hence the need for LDL in aging bodies decreases. This leads to increased production of LDL, as the body attempts to provide the building blocks for these hormones which are underused and so as we get older there is a higher quantity of LDL in circulation. This higher level of LDL increases the tendency for this substance to be deposited into the cell membranes where it can be oxidised to start the deadly sequelae of vessel-focussed cardiovascular disease. We have learned that oxidised LDL is a major contributor to cardiovascular disease in that it induces plaque formation and atherosclerosis.

Addressing excessive LDL in circulation

We have been told that among the chief functions of HDL is to clear LDL from circulation. Since excess LDL seems to be the heart attack substrate, the common view was that an increase in the levels of HDL would keep us safe. With this view, the drug company Pfizer spent 800 million dollars trying to develop an HDL-boosting medication. Unfortunately, this project was scrapped when the drug company learned that more people died on this drug than on placebo.

Additionally, since only 10%–25% of our body's cholesterol comes from our diet, logically we can't expect diet modification to make a significant impact on our cholesterol levels.

From the experience of Mr Fixx, an exercise fanatic, who wrote a book on running essentials and from all accounts appeared to be in good health yet collapsed and died of a heart attack at age 52, neither exercise, diet nor rising HDL levels appear to be able to save you. The question is: what can? We know that LDL is a major player, but how can we address this?

Statins are advertised to us as drugs which can inhibit the actions of HMG-CoA reductase, and should they work without the side effects, they could be an ideal approach to solving the challenges that an elevated LDL cause.

Unfortunately, these metabolic poisons, statins, are associated with a range of intolerable side effects, such as muscle spasms (pains), erectile dysfunction (in males), and a decrease in levels of acetyl coenzyme A, a molecule needed for normal cardiac function. Normal functional adults are converted to wheelchair users because of statins, so it is difficult to accept statins as the best option for treatment of LDL excess. In fact, it has been noted that patients on statins die earlier than patients not using statins. So, it has been concluded by some that statins will not save your life but may shorten it. With this understanding, therefore, it is safe to conclude that statins are not the best approach. Although the thought process is correct, the use of statins is not our best hope because of their side effect profile. Of interest, though, is that statins are derived from fungi; the question thus becomes: is there a substance in the plant world which may do what we are trying to do using statins without this horrible side effect profile?

The heart attack enzyme

HMG-CoA reductase is the enzyme which is primarily responsible for producing LDL in our bodies, both in our liver and in our intestine. Repeatedly, we have seen that when LDL levels rise, maybe through increased activity of HMG-CoA or the reduction of usage of LDL, there is an increased amount of circulating LDL with potentially disastrous consequences.

But this is not a straightforward process; there are triggers: why? I hear you ask. One never finds a youth without underlying health issues dying from a heart attack. But as we age the risk of this condition increases. The process seems to be that, with increasing age, the activity and level of HMG-CoA reductase fluctuate, as well as there is a reduced demand for LDL by our bodies, leading to increased levels of LDL cholesterol in circulation, which leads to the deposition of LDL into the cell membrane where it becomes oxidised, triggering a series of potential ill effects. It therefore appears that even if the HMG-CoA reductase is functioning normally, the reduced demand for LDL by our aging bodies can and will lead to an increase in circulating levels of LDL. The most sensible approach would therefore be the inhibition of the substance producing the LDL, that is the heart attack enzyme or HMG-CoA.

Heart attack enzyme busters!

These heart attack enzyme natural busters seemingly act in an identical manner to statins but without the horrendous side effects. Why then, I hear you ask, are these natural cholesterol busters not placed at the forefront in the fight against cholesterol and heart disease? The answer is simple: natural substances cannot be patented, thus presenting these natural substances as potential cholesterol busters would not be financially rewarding to drug companies.

The silk fruit

Since statins were extracted from fungi, which are plants, one wonders whether there exists a natural substance which can do the same as statins but without the horrendous side effects. In the silk fruit, one may have just found the semblance of an answer. The silk fruit is a plant that the silkworms eat to make silk. This mulberry fruit is also called a multiple fruit by some. The immature fruits are white, green, or pale yellow. In most species the fruit turns pink then red while ripening, then dark purple or black, and has a sweet flavour when fully ripe. These colourful berries can be eaten as fresh fruits or after they have been dried. They are found to be a good source of iron, vitamin C and several plant compounds, such as: anthocyanins, a family of antioxidants which may inhibit oxidation of LDL, thus helping to fight off cardiovascular disease; cyanidin, chlorogenic acid, again an antioxidant; rutin, a powerful antioxidant which protects against chronic conditions like cancer, diabetes and heart disease; and myricetin, a compound which may have protection against some cancers. Silk fruit extracts have been shown to lower cholesterol and blood sugar and reduce cancer risks.

The mechanism by which silk fruit is thought to produce its effect is through the inhibition of the heart attack enzyme, HMG-CoA, the exact same thing that statins are supposed to do but without the side effects.

In a recent study in which silk fruit was compared with statins, it was found that silk fruit was able to lower the levels of cholesterol to a greater degree than a commonly used statin.

Hibiscus

Hibiscus produces large, colourful flowers and has been used around the world as an herbal remedy. They are reported to have many health benefits, including reducing high blood pressure and high cholesterol. In one study focussing on patients with metabolic syndrome, hibiscus was found to lower blood sugar in these patients, as well as lower total cholesterol; simultaneously, it led to higher levels of HDL (good cholesterol) and improved insulin resistance, without the side effects of statins.

Garlic

This commonly used food seasoning appears to have more nutritional benefits than simply improving the taste of our meals. It is said that intake of a half to a whole clove of garlic per day lowers cholesterol levels approximately 10%. The mechanism is explained in terms of the garlic being able to decrease cholesterol absorption, and lower cholesterol and fatty acid synthesis. It therefore seems that garlic has a direct effect on the heart attack enzyme, but also has a secondary effect of decreasing cholesterol absorption.

Researchers tell us that it takes about eight weeks for garlic to lower cholesterol; also, it will take 4–12 weeks for 6 grams of garlic twice daily to decrease total cholesterol levels.

In garlic there is a compound called allicin which helps in thinning the blood and reduces the cholesterol levels. For this to be an effective cholesterol buster, it is believed that the garlic should be consumed raw and on an empty stomach. It is believed that cooking effectively dilutes the efficacy of allicin.

Foods rich in fibre

Foods like oatmeal, apples, bananas, prunes and beans are rich in soluble fibre which keeps your body from absorbing cholesterol. The impact of these foods may be mild since we only obtain 10%–25% of our total cholesterol from our diets, and these foods specifically reduce the quantity of cholesterol that is absorbed into our bodies.

Other useful foods

Plant sterols: plant sterols help to maintain healthy cholesterol levels because they help to limit the amount of cholesterol that is absorbed into our bodies whilst simultaneously, they can reduce the amount of cholesterol which our body produces. They have an inhibitory effect on the heart attack enzyme.

Red yeast rice

This describes a type of rice that has been fermented with yeast. It is believed that red yeast rice can reduce cholesterol because of its component monacolin K. Monacolins are able to reduce cholesterol production in our bodies by inhibiting the heart attack enzyme HMG-CoA (5-hydroxy-3-methylglutaryl-coenzyme A) reductase, the rate limiting step for cholesterol synthesis in the liver. The primary monacolin in red yeast rice is monacolin K, which has the same chemical structure as lovastatin. So why again did the drug companies think it necessary to produce this naturally occurring compound and rename it? This compound unfortunately has all the complications of statins, whilst monacolin K does not have these horrible side effects.

Bergamot

Bergamot, which is also referred to as Citrus bergamia, can reduce LDL and triglycerides while increasing HDL cholesterol. In one study, for example, it was shown that 500mg of bergamot can reduce bad cholesterol or LDL by 23% and increase good cholesterol by 25.9%. It is believed that bergamot can produce its effect because of its components, specifically neo hesperidin and naringin, which can bind with the heart attack enzyme, HMG-CoA reductase and so interrupt cholesterol production, leading to a reduction in cholesterol levels. Bergamot at an oral dose of 150–1000mg/day taken for 30–180 days will not only modulate total cholesterol, triglycerides, LDL and HDL, but also have a beneficial effect on body weight.

Niacin

Niacin lowers triglycerides by 25% and increases HDL (good cholesterol) by more than 30%. It may take a few weeks for niacin to alter cholesterol levels. Niacin is also known as vitamin B3 and plays a role in converting the foods we eat into energy by using fats and proteins.

Niacin is a B vitamin. When taken as a prescription in larger doses, it will help lower cholesterol and other fats in the bloodstream. It also raises the levels of HDL, or good cholesterol, as well as lowering the levels of LDL, the so-called bad cholesterol.

Niacin warning

Niacin has been associated with skin rashes and gastrointestinal problems and complicates the management of pre-existing diabetes; and though it does not cause diabetes, it increases the risk and brings it forward. Niacin in the form of nicotinamide has fewer side effects than nicotinic acid, but nicotinic acid is the form of niacin which lowers cholesterol. Other forms of niacin include nicotinamide and inositol nicotinate. Niacin is now no longer recommended by clinical guidelines to prevent cardiovascular disease.

Pause For Thought

- Is there a heart attack enzyme?
- Can any available substance neutralise the effect of this heart attack enzyme?
- Can silk fruit or hibiscus help in the neutralisation of this enzyme?
- Can food supplements such as garlic reduce or prevent the effect of the heart attack enzyme?
- Can foods rich in fibre reduce the effect of this heart attack enzyme?

Take Home Nuggets

- This heart attack enzyme functions in the production of cholesterol in the liver. This enzyme's function can be neutralised by many different substances among them are pharmacological substances as well as some non-pharmacological substances. Statins have been used but silk fruit, hibiscus, garlic and foods rick in fibre has shown some promise.

Notes

_____

_____

_____

_____

_____

_____

_____

_____

_____

_____

_____

_____

_____

_____

_____

_____

_____

_____

_____

_____

_____

_____

Notes

_____

_____

_____

_____

_____

_____

_____

_____

_____

_____

_____

_____

_____

_____

_____

_____

_____

_____

_____

_____

Chapter 13
Synopsis

- The role of the cardiovascular system
- Heart disease caused by dysfunction of the heart
- Management of this condition is based on its severity
- Acquired heart disease
- Vascular disease
- Oxidised cholesterol
- Need for a rethink
- Faulty use of statins
- Quality of life
- Pause For Thought
- Take Home Nuggets
- Pages for personal notes

The transfer of oxygen and nutrients to any location in the body is dependent on a pump mechanism, a transport medium or fluid and conduits through which that fluid flows. In animals the pump mechanism is the heart, the fluid is blood, and the conduits are the blood vessels. Cardiovascular disease is the result of dysfunction of any of the three modalities: the pump (heart), the fluid (blood) and the conduits (vessels), or various combinations of dysfunction in any of the components.

In our review of cardiovascular disease much effort was spent looking at the dysfunction in the blood vessels. Thus, cardiovascular disease includes the impact that may compromise the heart and thus its function (its ability to pump blood through the body), factors which affect the blood vessels, maybe by being broken or narrowed, and factors which may negatively affect the blood. If the carrying capacity of the blood to take nutrients and oxygen to various organs and tissues is compromised, that can also affect the cardiovascular system. It is believed that a drop in the blood haemoglobin by 1g/dL is an independent risk factor for cardiovascular morbidity and mortality.

Heart disease caused by dysfunction of the heart

This can be divided into: (1) congenital causes; and (2) acquired causes of heart disease. The congenital causes are related to developmental abnormality, leading to the abnormal heart even at birth. The heart may lack all its distinct chambers, there may be problems with the valves, either because the valves do not effectively prevent the blood in the various chambers from mixing, or the partition between both sides of the heart may be undeveloped.

Management of this condition is based on its severity

In very severe cases, surgery is considered just after birth. In the milder cases medications may be considered to bring about closure of the heart defect even after birth. Alternatively, in its mildest form cautious observation is preferred.

Acquired heart disease

This type of heart disease develops because of the insults to which our hearts are subjected, maybe through exposure to various toxins. Among a variety of chemicals used to treat cancer which have spread over the body are some referred to as alkylating agents. These agents are known to destroy the very cells which make up the heart, thus making our hearts weaker.

Another group of agents called angiogenesis inhibitors cause heart changes resulting from diminished oxygen supply; this leads to ischaemia and dysfunction of the heart.

A third group of chemotherapeutic agents called anthracyclines produce free radicals which function in weakening the heart muscles, leading to left ventricular dysfunction, and hence compromise the ability of the heart to pump blood around our bodies.

So, these agents have a direct ill effect on the functioning of the heart. These drugs are mainly used in patients with metastatic cancers.

Social drugs like tobacco have a more indirect effect on the heart. Cigarette smoking thickens blood, increasing the risk of blood clot formation and atherosclerosis or narrowing of blood vessels, reducing blood supply to various organs and tissues. If the blood supply to the heart is reduced, there will be chest pains and ischaemic changes in the heart, resulting in weakening of the heart.

Cocaine use leads to higher blood pressure and damage to the structure of the heart which may lead to abnormal beats, chest pains, congestive heart failure and even death.

Vascular disease

Vascular disease can be either inherited or acquired.

Much of the discussion in this book has been focussed on the acquired types of vascular disease and the causation of atherosclerosis. We have spoken at length about the effect of cholesterol and its vessel narrowing impact. This causes increased blood pressure and may lead to pain on walking, as well as formation of blood clots which can travel in the bloodstream and may completely cut off blood supply to various organs and tissues. If this occurs in the heart, the result is a heart attack; in the brain the result is a stroke; in the kidneys, kidney failure. In the lower limbs there will be pain, discolouration of the affected limb, and swelling. Eventually, gangrene will set in, and a lifesaving amputation of the affected limb becomes necessary.

Cardiovascular disease is the result of multifactorial causes, and treating this condition successfully is therefore challenging. Current thinking suggests that cardiovascular disease is generally caused by insults on the vasculature which led to impairment in the blood supply to various organs and tissues. The current teaching suggests that the insult on the vasculature is largely contributed to by progressive narrowing of the blood vessels, a condition called atherosclerosis. With the progressive narrowing of the blood vessels, there is a reduction in blood supply to organs and tissues downstream. It is believed that the progressive narrowing of the vessels is largely caused by the deposition of LDL cholesterol into the vessel wall which becomes oxidised and forms plaque. It is believed that the insult to the blood vessels wall is directly related to the levels of homocysteine in circulation. Homocysteine is an amino acid which is derived from another amino acid called methionine, which is present in all animal and plant proteins. This homocysteine is needed to repair the walls of the blood vessels, and it is the occasional excess levels of homocysteine which have a direct relationship with cardiovascular disease.

We have, however, seen many conditions which directly or indirectly affect the normal functioning of the heart. We also note that there are several underlying diseases which affect the normal functioning of the heart: diseases such as diabetes, high blood pressure, hormonal dysfunction, metabolic syndrome, or syndrome X all influence the normal functioning of the heart. We have seen, though, that the incidence of cardiovascular disease is on the rise, and the deaths resulting from this disease are still too high.

Granted, we have made some progress with specialist centres, minimally invasive procedures, multidisciplinary teams a wider range of medications and more pointed investigations.

Why do we continue to see a rise in the incidence of this condition despite all our efforts? Are we missing appropriate steps to give us better results?

Oxidised cholesterol

Though we are lectured repeatedly about the effects of cholesterol, and almost as candies cholesterol-lowering drugs are prescribed daily, yet a significant dent is not being made in the incidence of the disease process. Are we navigating along the wrong path? Many have argued that individuals die of cardiovascular disease with normal cholesterol levels, though cholesterol-lowering drugs called statins are regularly prescribed.

It has been increasingly realised that statins will not cause you to live longer, and studies show that statins can reduce your lifespan.

Statins are metabolic poisons, the use of which we may be wise to reconsider, in light of the frequency with which they are prescribed, their side effect profile and their apparent failure to prolong life.

Individuals have been shown to lose their ability to walk and be confined to wheelchairs, experience severe muscle cramps, irregular heartbeats, erectile dysfunction, reduction in the levels of some essential hormones, and show and experience features of premature aging.

Need for a rethink

We know that 75–90% of the total cholesterol in our bodies is produced in our livers; it would therefore seem that cholesterol plays a meaningful role in our bodies. It is involved in making the sex hormones, stress hormones and vitamin D, and in the formation of cell membranes. It is easy to conclude that cholesterol is not bad since it performs such a vital role. Yet our management is heavily focussed on reducing our cholesterol levels with unpleasant side effects. Must we rethink our screening methods? It would seem obvious since individuals still succumb to heart disease even with a normal lipid profile. Once there is a suspicion of cardiovascular disease there is almost a knee-jerk reaction initiated with the request for a lipid profile test and the commencement of statins. The lipid profile test, however, fails to measure the most insidious form of cholesterol, oxidised LDL cholesterol. Oxidised LDL cholesterol is known to be atherosclerotic and induces plaque formation, yet routinely we do not test for the levels of oxidised LDL. If we do not screen for the major culprit, we are obviously unable to treat the condition appropriately. Additionally, the level of homocysteine is not routinely screened for, but we know there is a direct relationship between the levels of homocysteine and cardiovascular disease.

There is an available screening test to determine the levels of oxidised LDL, albeit this test is not widely available, so our efforts should be more focussed on making this test more widely available; this, coupled with homocysteine levels, may give a more accurate determination of those at risk of a major cardiovascular event. Additionally, there is the non-invasive screening test called the carotid intermediary wall thickness (CIMT) which is a simple ultrasound scan of the carotid artery wall thickness that allows one to determine the degree of wall thickness and hence plaque build-up in the vessel. This non-invasive screening test can also be used to determine the success of your treatment. Blood tests are useful but can be imperfect. Additionally, a CT scan can be performed, a specialised study called the electron beam computed tomography (EBCT). These scans examine the abdominal cavity and chest with the capacity to visualise the coronary arteries. In this way they can detect coronary artery disease and other abnormalities, including tumours and aneurysms in the chest, abdomen, and pelvis. Having these scans even in the absence of symptoms allows for the detection of abnormalities before symptoms appear.

The EBCT can be conducted within 10–15 minutes and, unlike other CT scans and MRI, this investigation is conducted in an open environment and allows for a quick, three-dimensional assessment of the heart, lungs, and blood vessels.

The EBCT scan can be used to determine the extent of calcium build-up in the lining of arteries inclusive of the coronary arteries. A paper published in the American Journal of Epidemiology has shown correlation between the degree of calcification and the degree of atherosclerosis in the arteries. Simply put, a low level of calcium build-up in arteries means that your risk of coronary artery disease is low. A high-level means that you are at a higher risk of cardiovascular problems in the future.

The major concern with this test is the degree of radiation exposure which can be as high as ten times more than that of a standard X-ray. Radiation is a risk factor for the development of some types of cancer. The EBCT is also associated with false positive results. An area of suspicion requiring further investigation may show up in this investigation, which on further review is an innocent finding or no lesion is found. Nonetheless, if the results are normal, it can delay further screening by five to ten years.

The faulty use of statins

In the UK there are five statins which have been approved for use to lower cholesterol; in the USA there are at least seven such preparations, all of which are supposedly doing the same thing. They seem to inhibit HMG-CoA reductase, an enzyme which plays an integral role in the liver synthesis of cholesterol and is the heart attack enzyme. As we have said repeatedly above, 75-90% of our body's cholesterol is made in the liver, and we get only 10%–25% of cholesterol from our diets. The practice of using statins to lower cholesterol may be misadvised. It is now apparent that our focus should be preventing LDL cholesterol in our blood vessel walls from becoming oxidised.

Quality of life

Above we have referenced the ill effects on our heart with the use of certain classes of chemotherapeutic drugs to treat cancer patients. If there is evidence which supports the direct effect of these agents on the heart, should we not also be concerned about the effect of these agents on the resultant quality of life of the recipient? Surely this needs to be a major consideration about not only the anticancer preparations, but also the widespread use of statins with their history of crippling side effects.

Logic tells us that though LDL is necessary in our bodies to produce sex hormones, cortisol, and vitamin D, and it plays an integral role in cell membrane structure and repair, at higher levels, the risk of it being oxidised is increased, and it is in this oxidised state LDL is able to produce its most deleterious effect on the cardiovascular system. The rationale for statins, therefore, is sensible, but as indicated in Chapter 12, there are other naturally occurring substitutes which produce identical effects to statins but without the disgusting, horrible side effects seen with statins. Like homocysteine, an amino acid which plays an integral role in the repair of blood vessels, when the levels are too high it has a deleterious effect on cardiovascular health. We have learned that some dietary supplements are able to reduce the levels of homocysteine in our bodies. Unlike homocysteine, a product of the amino acid methionine, which is present in all plant and animal proteins, our bodies only obtain 10%–25% of its cholesterol from the foods we eat, so reduction of our cholesterol intake through the foods we consume may not reduce our cholesterol load significantly, and so there is a need for supplements which effectively reduce our cholesterol production while limiting the total amount of cholesterol absorbed from our foods. This must be our focus if we are to neutralise the effects of cholesterol on our population.

Pause For Thought

- Can diseases of the heart lead to cardiovascular disease?
- Can vessel disease lead to cardiovascular disease?
- Can the transported fluid cause cardiovascular disease?

Take Home Nuggets

- Cardiovascular disease is multifactorial and each of its components can become dysfunctional leading to cardiovascular disease. The pump or heart may be dysfunctional because of a congenital defect, or in the case of the acquired variety because of an insult. The vessels dysfunction can also lead to cardiovascular disease. Again, these vessels can be congenitally dysfunctional or become dysfunctional because of exposure to different insults. The fluid transported in the vessels can also cause cardiovascular disease. The fluid could develop these changes because of some genetic condition or because it was acquired because of life style factors or because of dehydration.

Notes

Notes

_____

_____

_____

_____

_____

_____

_____

_____

_____

_____

_____

_____

_____

_____

_____

_____

_____

_____

_____

_____

_____

_____

Epilogue

Reclaiming your health is not only possible but necessary if you want to add years to your life and life to your years. Let us explore how this is possible. We look at the 9 most common chronic health issues of today and indicate how these can be overcome. We will explore the disease process, trying to understand their causation, and determine through reliable scientific research how to keep these health challenges at bay. We will also delve into common-sense practices which will play invaluable roles in rendering the disease dormant and in some cases completely reverse the disease process. We encourage the employment of various common-sense measures, as well as provide evidence on how the advised measures work. We are strong proponents of social and preventative medicine and recognise the failure of traditional approaches in the fight against a variety of disease processes.

In this series of 12 books, we will produce easy-to-read manuscripts about each of the nine most common chronic medical conditions, and a book on women's health after the menopause, as well as a book on men's health in which we will question the issue of andropause and address some of the challenges of getting more advanced in age.

With experience and training in organic chemistry, biochemistry and medicine, both as a clinical practitioner and as a trainer for in excess of 30 years, coupled with my years of teaching, I believe that I am uniquely positioned to help you add years to your life and life to your years by attacking and overcoming the vices of modern living which have almost succeeded in overcoming and burdening our very existence through these nine most common chronic ailments. The last three books in this series not only address the issues of getting older, but also suggest methods which you can employ to present the most active versions of yourself even in your twilight years. The final book in this series was empowered by my stem cell research, the legal and ethical issues, during the preparation and fulfilment for the master's degree in law which I was able to complete.

Notes

Notes

www.ingramcontent.com/pod-product-compliance
Lightning Source LLC
Chambersburg PA
CBHW081815200326
41597CB00023B/4259